Interventional Vascular Radiology

and

Interventional Neurovascular Radiology

A Report of the National Confidential Enquiry into Perioperative Deaths

Data collection period
1 April 1998 to 31 March 1999

Compiled by:

K G Callum MS FRCS

F Whimster MHM

Published 21 November 2000 by the National Confidential Enquiry into Perioperative Deaths

35-43 Lincoln's Inn Fields, London WC2A 3PN
Tel: (020) 7831 6430
Fax: (020) 7430 2958
Email: info@ncepod.org.uk
Website: www.ncepod.org.uk

Requests for further information should be addressed to the Chief Executive

ISBN   0 9522069 8 6

A company limited by guarantee   Company number   3019382
Registered charity number   1075588

This report is printed on paper produced from wood pulp originating from managed sustainable plantations and is chlorine-free, acid-free, recyclable and biodegradable.

Additional information

This report is available for downloading from the NCEPOD website at www.ncepod.org.uk

Copies can also be purchased from the NCEPOD office.

The analysis of data from questionnaires is not included in full
in this report. A supplement containing additional data, and copies of
the questionnaires, is available free of charge from the NCEPOD office.

A 010929

WG 500

NATIONAL CEPOD

ACKNOWLEDGEMENTS

This report could not have been achieved without the support and cooperation of a wide range of individuals and organisations. Our particular thanks go to the following:

- The Royal College of Radiologists and the British Society of Interventional Radiologists for supporting the concept of this study.

- The Local Reporters, whose names are listed in Appendices D and E.

- All those radiologists whose names are listed in Appendices F and G, who contributed to the Enquiry by completing questionnaires.

- The Advisors whose names are listed overleaf.

- Those bodies, whose names are listed in Appendix B, who provide the funding to cover the cost of the Enquiry, together with the Department of Health who provided additional support.

- Mr Chris Macklin, Surgical Registrar, Derbyshire Royal Infirmary, for the illustrations on the front cover.

The Steering Group, Clinical Coordinators and Chief Executive would also like to record their appreciation of the hard work and tolerance of the NCEPOD administrative staff: Peter Allison, Fatima Chowdhury, Paul Coote, Sheree Cornwall, Jennifer Drummond and Dolores Jarman.

The views expressed in this publication are those of NCEPOD and not necessarily those of the National Institute for Clinical Excellence, or any other funding body.

NATIONAL **CEPOD**

CLINICAL CONTRIBUTORS

NCEPOD COORDINATOR

K G Callum   Clinical Coordinator, NCEPOD and Consultant General and Vascular Surgeon, Derbyshire Royal Infirmary

SPECIALTY ADVISORS

Interventional vascular radiology

J Dyet   Hull Royal Infirmary and Royal College of Radiologists' representative on NCEPOD Steering Group

P A Gaines   Northern General Hospital, Sheffield

I Gillespie   Royal Infirmary of Edinburgh

L C Johnston   Belfast City Hospital

M Ruttley   University Hospital of Wales (retired)

Interventional neurovascular radiology

A Gholkar   Newcastle General Hospital

A J Molyneux   The Radcliffe Infirmary, Oxford

CONTENTS

NATIONAL CEPOD

TABLES, FIGURES AND QUESTIONS

1 Interventional Vascular Radiology

General data analysis

Patient profile

Specialty and experience of the medical team

Facilities, personnel and monitoring

Complications

Postmortem examinations

2 Interventional Neurovascular Radiology

General data analysis

Patient profile

Facilities, personnel and monitoring

Complications

Postmortem examinations

 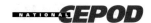

FOREWORD

Significant advances in interventional techniques, particularly in vascular and neurovascular radiology, in the last decade have led NCEPOD to explore the morbidity and mortality associated with such procedures. It should be appreciated that this is a new area of investigation, but in view of the frequency with which these minimally invasive techniques are being carried out, it is important that the consequences of such interventions should be investigated. Furthermore, this is an area of team working which has developed very significantly, the relationships between members of that team and the role that each play are highlighted in an investigation of this type. There is a need to understand the potential roles that each member of the team can play and the responsibilities that each should take at different stages in the care of the patient.

It is fundamental to the development of new techniques that adequate facilities should be available. What is highlighted in this report, therefore, is the necessity for interventional radiologists and surgeons to have not only sufficient experience and expertise, but also the facilities and equipment with which to carry out their tasks in as safe an environment as possible.

This report not only highlights the frequency with which these procedures are now being carried out, but also the safety of such techniques, recognising that the patients in question are frequently seriously ill, such that minor complications could have various serious outcomes. This is reflected in the very low mortality rate of around 2%. The fact that these patients are so severely ill links with this year's general NCEPOD report "Then and Now" in emphasising the need for both high dependency and intensive care facilities to be available where such clinical activities are being performed.

The increasing demand for interventional procedures of this type is as yet unmet by the number of consultant vascular radiologists and neurovascular radiologists who are available to satisfy that need. This report, therefore, further highlights the need for an increase in resources which is emphasised in our report "Then and Now" also published this year.

John Ll Williams
Chairman

NATIONAL CEPOD

1 INTERVENTIONAL VASCULAR RADIOLOGY

RECOMMENDATIONS

- It is essential that vascular radiologists and surgeons work together as a team both in the decision as to what procedures to undertake and in the management of any complications (pages 13-14, 20, 22).

- The interventional radiologist needs to have sufficient experience, facilities and equipment to perform the procedure safely and to deal with any complications which may arise (pages 14-18, 20).

- Monitoring of pulse oximetry, blood pressure and ECG should be performed during all interventional radiology procedures; this should be done by someone other than the radiologist performing the procedure (page 17).

- Cannulation of the femoral artery should always be below the inguinal ligament to avoid the danger of retroperitoneal haematoma. Medical and nursing staff must be aware of the risks of this serious complication in order to act early when necessary (pages 19-20).

- Thrombolytic therapy should be used with caution, especially in the elderly (over 75 years) who are more prone to cerebral haemorrhage. Patients with thrombolysis continuing after they have left the radiology department should be nursed in a high dependency unit so that complications may be diagnosed and treated without delay (pages 21-22).

1. INTERVENTIONAL VASCULAR RADIOLOGY

INTRODUCTION

With the availability of new and smaller devices over the last 20 years, interventional vascular radiology has become increasingly important in the treatment of blood vessel related diseases. The interventional procedure is attractive to both doctors and patients because it is performed under local anaesthesia and the insertion of the device is done by direct needle puncture through the skin without surgical incision. It may be used to treat a wide variety of conditions, but the common theme is that a fine catheter is inserted into a blood vessel and, by the use of imaging (usually X-ray) and a guidewire, narrow areas in blood vessels may be stretched (balloon angioplasty) or held open (stent); used to deliver a drug to dissolve blood clot (thrombolysis); used to insert a central venous catheter to deliver chemotherapy or intravenous nutrition or for haemodialysis; used to occlude vessels with small particles to stop bleeding in inaccessible sites (embolisation); used to place a filter to allow blood through, but not to allow blood clot to pass (inferior vena cava filter); or used to make a new connection between the portal and systemic circulation in portal hypertension (TIPS).

As these procedures can be done under local anaesthetic, usually with minimal upset to the patient, less fit patients can be treated, who would not be well enough to undergo a formal surgical operation. Inevitably, therefore, some of these patients are going to die from their underlying disease following, for example, an angioplasty which in many of the patients is an incident in the course of their disease. However, because many of these patients are already very ill, otherwise minor complications may have very serious consequences.

DATA COLLECTION

Data were requested from all NHS hospitals undertaking these procedures in England, Scotland, Wales, Northern Ireland, Guernsey and Jersey. Participation was voluntary and some hospitals chose, for a variety of reasons, not to participate.

Information on the total number of patients undergoing interventional radiology procedures on a monthly basis, together with notification of any deaths occurring within 30 days of the procedure, were collected for the period 1 April 1998 - 31 March 1999.

GENERAL DATA ANALYSIS

Monthly returns of procedures performed

One hundred and sixty-two hospitals initially agreed to participate in the study, although this reduced to 154 who subsequently contributed monthly data. Each hospital was required to send in a monthly return of all patients undergoing interventional vascular radiological procedures in the hospital. A total of 1848 forms should therefore have been received. The return of monthly data is shown in Figure 1.1.

A regional breakdown of the number of monthly forms received is given in Table 1.1. The return rate of monthly forms was commendably high; the rate of 72% from Scotland was a little disappointing and may have been due to similar studies being conducted simultaneously in that country.

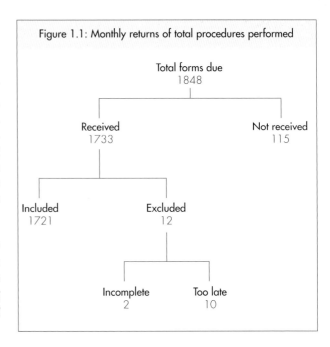

Figure 1.1: Monthly returns of total procedures performed

Total forms due
1848

Received
1733

Not received
115

Included
1721

Excluded
12

Incomplete
2

Too late
10

Region	Number of participating hospitals	Monthly forms received	Monthly forms expected	Return rate
Anglia & Oxford	12	144	144	100%
North Thames	12	132	144	92%
North West	21	243	252	96%
Northern & Yorkshire	19	213	228	93%
South & West	17	180	204	88%
South Thames	19	215	228	94%
Trent	15	165	180	92%
West Midlands	16	183	192	95%
Wales	10	120	120	100%
Northern Ireland	2	24	24	100%
Scotland	9	78	108	72%
Guernsey	1	12	12	100%
Jersey	1	12	12	100%
Total	154	1721	1848	94%

Table 1.1: Monthly returns by region

Reported procedures

This is the first study where NCEPOD has been able to collect data on the total number of procedures performed, as well as details of those patients who died. Just over 21 000 (21 112) of these procedures were reported by the 154 participating hospitals in the year from 1 April 1998 to 31 March 1999, giving a mean of 137 procedures per centre.

Reported deaths

Figure 1.2 shows that a total of 511 reports of deaths within 30 days of a procedure were received, reducing to 476 when 35 inappropriate reports were excluded (Table 1.2), giving a mortality rate of just over 2% (476/21 112; 2.3%).

A further 25 reports were received after the deadline of 31 August 1999 and 6 remained incomplete despite all efforts to identify missing information, leaving 445 cases for inclusion in the study.

A regional breakdown of the remaining 445 deaths is shown in Table 1.3.

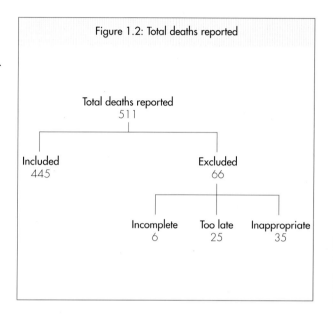

Figure 1.2: Total deaths reported

Total deaths reported
511

Included 445

Excluded 66

Incomplete 6

Too late 25

Inappropriate 35

Table 1.2: Inappropriate reports received and excluded	
Reason for exclusion	Number
More than 30 days *(day of procedure to day of death)*	19
Duplicate report	2
Procedure excluded by NCEPOD criteria	9
Procedure performed in non-participating independent hospital	4
Death outside study period	5
Total	**35**

Table 1.3: Deaths reported to NCEPOD by region	
Region	Deaths reported
Anglia & Oxford	35
North Thames	68
North West	49
Northern & Yorkshire	67
South & West	68
South Thames	29
Trent	40
West Midlands	36
Wales	13
Northern Ireland	1
Scotland	39
Guernsey	0
Jersey	0
Total	**445**

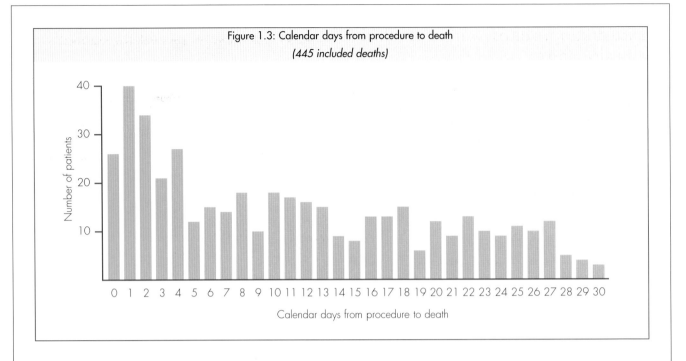

Figure 1.3: Calendar days from procedure to death
(445 included deaths)

Figure 1.3 shows the distribution of the number of calendar days between procedure (day 0) and death. The fact that the number of days from procedure to death was so widely distributed suggests that most patients died for reasons unrelated to the procedure.

Figure 1.4 shows the distribution of age and sex.

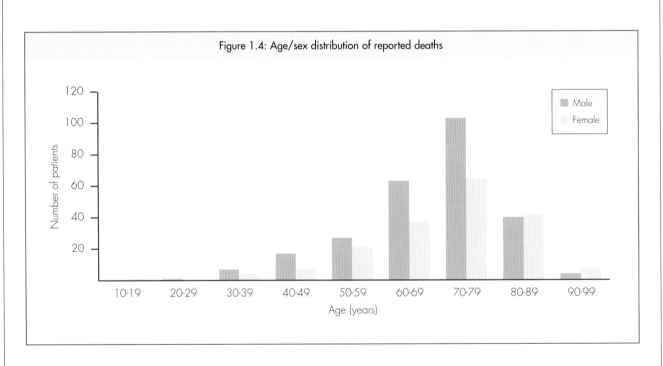

Figure 1.4: Age/sex distribution of reported deaths

Distribution, return and analysis of questionnaires

Questionnaires were sent to the consultant radiologist responsible for the care of each of the 445 patients included. Figure 1.5 shows the return and analysis rates of questionnaires sent.

Table 1.4: Reasons for exclusion of questionnaires from analysis	
Reason for exclusion	Number
Questionnaire received too late	11
Questionnaire incomplete	2
Questionnaire completed for wrong procedure	1
Total	14

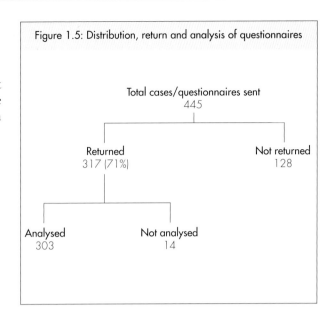

Figure 1.5: Distribution, return and analysis of questionnaires

Total cases/questionnaires sent
445

Returned
317 (71%)

Not returned
128

Analysed
303

Not analysed
14

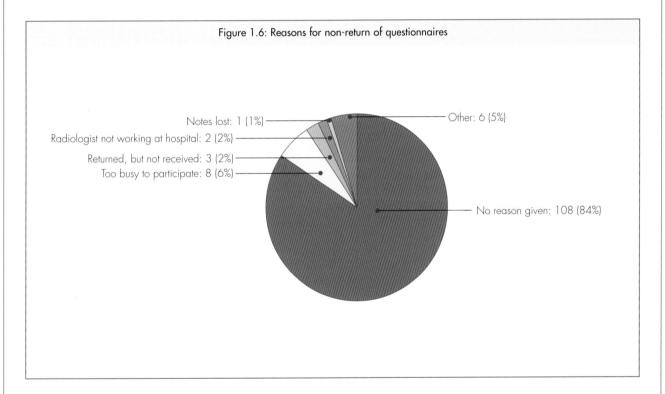

Figure 1.6: Reasons for non-return of questionnaires

Notes lost: 1 (1%)
Radiologist not working at hospital: 2 (2%)
Returned, but not received: 3 (2%)
Too busy to participate: 8 (6%)
Other: 6 (5%)
No reason given: 108 (84%)

In the majority of cases (84%) where no questionnaire was returned, no reason was offered for an inability to do so. In three cases the radiologist indicated that the questionnaire had been returned although it was not received in the NCEPOD offices.

Table 1.5: Regional distribution, return and analysis rates				
Region	Questionnaires distributed	Questionnaires returned	Return rate	Questionnaires analysed
Anglia & Oxford	35	31	89%	30
North Thames	68	22	32%	20
North West	49	37	76%	37
Northern & Yorkshire	67	55	82%	55
South & West	68	55	81%	54
South Thames	29	15	52%	15
Trent	40	32	80%	29
West Midlands	36	29	81%	29
Wales	13	11	85%	11
Northern Ireland	1	1	100%	1
Scotland	39	29	74%	22
Total	445	317	71%	303

Table 1.5 shows the return rates by region and the majority of these were in excess of 80%; of note were the disappointingly low return rates of South Thames (52%) and, in particular, North Thames where only one third (32%) of questionnaires were returned.

Procedures

Tables 1.6, 1.7 and 1.8 summarise the total number of procedures performed, together with deaths, for arterial, venous and other interventions respectively.

Table 1.6: Endovascular interventions (arterial)												
Intervention	Angioplasty		Stent		Thrombolysis		Atherectomy		Embolisation		Aneurysm exclusion	
Site	Total	Deaths	Total	Deaths	Total	Deaths	Total	Deaths	Total	Deaths	Total	Deaths
Carotid (includes internal & external)	18	-	57	1 (2%)	4	-	-	-	29	-	3	-
Brachiocephalic	13	-	8	-	10	-	-	-	4	-	-	-
Subclavian	103	-	50	-	23	2 (9%)	-	-	19	-	1	-
Other	27	1 (4%)	6	-	14	2 (14%)	-	-	298	4 (1%)	1	-
Gut	20	1 (5%)	18	1 (6%)	-	-	-	-	149	7 (5%)	2	-
Renal	408	5 (1%)	322	5 (2%)	6	-	-	-	214	3 (1%)	-	-
Aorta	71	-	73	-	6	-	-	-	2	-	3	-
Iliac	3619	31 (1%)	1208	8 (1%)	134	5 (4%)	13	-	31	-	8	-
Pelvic	70	1 (1%)	6	-	6	-	-	-	236	6 (3%)	2	-
Femoral	5680	47 (1%)	76	-	550	17 (3%)	11	-	33	1 (3%)	10	-
Popliteal	1101	15 (1%)	8	-	153	8 (5%)	-	-	3	-	1	-
Tibial	526	9 (2%)	1	-	41	-	-	-	20	-	1	-
Graft	219	-	6	-	227	17 (7%)	5	-	3	-	-	-
Pulmonary	-	-	1	-	11	1 (9%)	-	-	31	-	-	-
Total	11 875	110 (1%)	1840	15 (1%)	1185	52 (4%)	29	-	1072	21 (2%)	32	-

Intervention Site	Angioplasty		Stent		Thrombolysis		Embolisation	
	Total	Deaths	Total	Deaths	Total	Deaths	Total	Deaths
Brachiocephalic	47	-	26	-	16	-	-	-
Subclavian	63	-	32	-	26	1 (4%)	1	-
Superior vena cava	15	1 (7%)	266	17 (6%)	17	2 (12%)	1	-
Inferior vena cava	2	-	16	2 (13%)	3	-	-	-
Hepatic	9	-	25	-	-	-	11	-
Portal	43	-	13	-	1	-	13	-
Graft	48	-	3	-	15	-	-	-
Renal	3	-	3	-	1	-	4	-
Iliac	10	-	14	-	15	-	19	-
Infrainguinal	7	-	1	-	3	1 (33%)	15	-
Gonadal	-	-	-	-	-	-	491	-
Total	247	1 (<1%)	399	19 (5%)	97	4 (4%)	555	-

Table 1.7: Endovascular interventions (venous)

The two most common venous procedures were gonadal vein embolisation, which is performed for varicocoele and has made operation for this condition a rarity, and superior vena cava (SVC) stent placement, performed to relieve swelling of the upper half of the body due to oedema caused by obstruction of the SVC, usually due to intrathoracic malignancy.

Table 1.8: Other interventions

Intervention	Total	Deaths	
Central venous access (not temporary)	3052	36	(1%)
Foreign body	70	1	(1%)
Inferior vena cava filters	501	17	(3%)
Transjugular intrahepatic portosystemic shunt (TIPS)	158	27	(17%)
Total	3781	81	(2%)

In 35 cases death was considered to be related to the procedure and in 13 of these the advisors thought that the risk of complications related to the procedure was justified bearing in mind the very serious medical condition of the patient. Thus, technical problems where the procedure contributed to the death of the patient occurred in 22 cases (0.1%) or about one in 1000 cases. While this indicates a very high standard of care it still leaves some room for improvement. Details of these problems will be discussed in later sections of this report, together with recommendations for improvement. There were also a number of instances where it was felt that care could have been better, even though patients did not suffer as a result, and these too will be discussed.

PATIENT PROFILE

The report hereafter deals only with those patients who died.

Key Point

• *Interventional vascular radiology procedures are generally safe with around 21 000 procedures performed in participating hospitals during the year and 476 deaths (2%). Many of these patients were extremely unwell and not fit enough for open surgery.*

Urgency of procedure

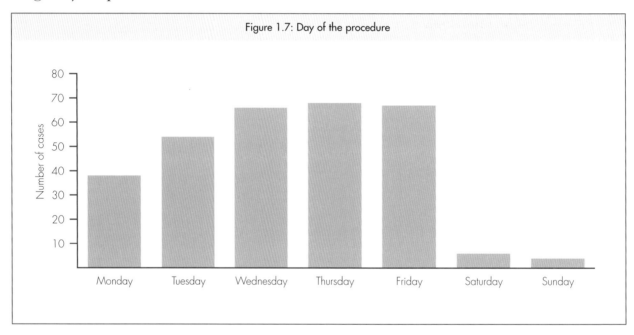

Figure 1.7: Day of the procedure

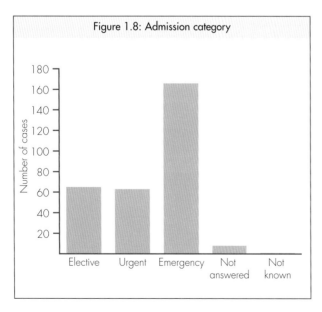

Figure 1.8: Admission category

The majority of procedures appear to be done midweek, with less on a Monday and very few performed at a weekend. It is interesting to note, however, that although the majority of interventional vascular procedures were performed electively, of those who died a large number were done urgently (63/303; 21%) or as an emergency (166/303; 55%).

Fitness of the patient

This was assessed using the American Society of Anesthesiologists (ASA) Classification of Physical Status:

ASA 1   a normal healthy patient.

ASA 2   a patient with mild systemic disease.

ASA 3   a patient with severe systemic disease that limits activity but is not incapacitating.

ASA 4   a patient with incapacitating systemic disease that is a constant threat to life.

ASA 5   a moribund patient not expected to survive for 24 hours with or without an operation.

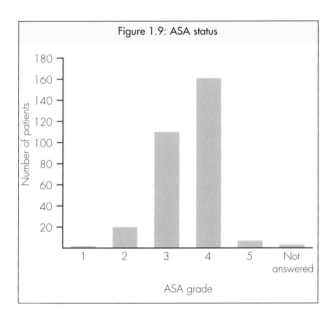

Figure 1.9: ASA status

Table 1.9: Coexisting medical problems (268 cases; answers may be multiple)	
Coexisting medical problem	Number
Cardiac	153
Respiratory	93
Vascular	81
Diabetes mellitus	76
Malignancy	62
Renal	57
Gastrointestinal	48
Sepsis	43
Neurological	38
Haematological	37
Nutritional	19
Alcohol-related problems	16
Musculoskeletal	15
Obesity	13
Psychiatric	10
Other endocrine	8
Genetic abnormality	1
Other	15

Table 1.9 gives further confirmation of the considerable extent to which patients who died following interventional radiology had a number of other coexisting medical problems.

The majority (278/303; 92%) of those patients who died following interventional vascular radiology had severe systemic disease (ASA grade 3 or higher). Many of these patients would not have been considered fit enough for open surgery.

Coexisting problems (other than the main diagnosis) existed in 268/303 (88%) of the patients and these are shown in Table 1.9. In only 29/297 (10%) cases where the question was answered did the patient have no coexisting medical problems.

Table 1.10: Anticipated risk of death related to the proposed procedure	
Risk of death	Number
Not expected	163
Small but significant	76
Definite risk	50
Expected	7
Not answered	7
Total	303

There were seven patients who had vascular interventions even though they were expected to die (Table 1.10). Two were for the relief of very unpleasant symptoms:

CASE 1 • A 58-year-old patient with lung cancer in whom embolisation was performed to stop his distressing, severe recurrent haemoptysis.

CASE 2 • A 55-year-old patient with distressing swelling of the face and arms, together with breathlessness due to superior vena cava (SVC) obstruction caused by squamous carcinoma of the lung. She had previously had a successful stent which had then thrombosed and thrombolysis was given to try and clear the stent and relieve her unpleasant symptoms.

In a further two cases the intervention was a 'last ditch' attempt to save life:

CASE 3 • A 76-year-old patient who had persistent severe bleeding following a transurethral prostatectomy. Embolisation of the internal iliac artery was performed to try and stop bleeding. The radiologist thought that there would have been a better chance of the patient surviving had the urologist called for help earlier.

CASE 4 • An 89-year-old patient having revision of a recurrent fractured neck of femur developed very heavy bleeding which had proved impossible to control surgically, so embolisation of the profunda femoris was performed. This was technically successful but sadly by this time the patient had developed a coagulopathy.

There were a further two patients with persistent pulmonary emboli despite adequate anticoagulation:

CASE 5 • A 64-year-old patient with multiple pulmonary emboli had sudden deterioration due to a further pulmonary embolus confirmed on spiral CT. He had already survived a previous massive pulmonary embolism so it was thought worth trying a caval filter to prevent further emboli. This was believed to be his only hope, as he would not have survived a pulmonary embolectomy.

CASE 6 • A 51-year-old patient with multiple pulmonary emboli who, despite anticoagulation, was in respiratory distress. It was felt that there was a small chance of recovery if further pulmonary emboli could be prevented and an IVC filter was inserted.

Lastly, thrombolysis was tried in a relatively young man who was not fit enough to withstand an operation:

CASE 7 • A 45-year-old patient with acute on chronic aortoiliac occlusion. He was not considered fit enough to survive surgery because of severe ischaemic heart disease. Death was expected because of the severe extent of his ischaemia, and thrombolysis was thought to be the only hope of restoring the circulation and giving him a chance of survival. The fact that there was no ICU or HDU bed did not help in this patient's management and he subsequently died of pulmonary oedema due to congestive cardiac failure (see also page 18).

Each of these cases was reviewed by the vascular radiology advisors and was considered to be justifiable either in the relief of symptoms or because there was a very small chance of the patient surviving a procedure that would cause very little upset to them.

SPECIALTY AND EXPERIENCE OF THE MEDICAL TEAM

Specialty of the clinical team

Tables 1.11 and 1.12 show the specialty of the consultants under whose care the patients were at the time of their procedure.

Table 1.11: Specialty of consultant surgeon under whose care the patient was at the time of the procedure	
Specialty	Number
General	2
General with interest in vascular surgery	97
General with interest in gastroenterology	18
General with interest in urology	1
General with interest in endocrinology	1
General with interest in breast surgery	1
General with interest in hepatobiliary surgery	1
General with interest in thoracic surgery	1
Vascular	46
Urology	3
Gynaecology	2
Orthopaedic	2
Transplantation	2
Cardiac/thoracic/cardiothoracic	1
Oral/maxillofacial	1
Oncology	1

Table 1.12: Specialty of consultant physician under whose care the patient was at the time of the procedure	
Specialty	Number
General with interest in gastroenterology	16
General with interest in renal medicine	8
General with interest in thoracic medicine	6
General with interest in endocrinology	5
General with interest in cardiology	3
General with interest in rheumatology	2
General with interest in paediatrics	1
Gastroenterology	11
Renal medicine	9
Haematology	9
Thoracic medicine	8
Care of the elderly	8
Oncology	6
Endocrinology	3
Cardiology	2
Radiotherapy	1
Pulmonary oncology	1
Palliative care	1

Almost all patients were under the care of the appropriate specialist, such as vascular patients under the care of the vascular surgeons and the patients having TIPS under the care of gastroenterologists. However, there were a few exceptions:

CASE 8 • *A 55-year-old patient who was referred by a nephrologist for dilatation of popliteal arterial stenosis. This occluded two days later and the patient was not seen by a vascular surgeon until too late and an amputation was subsequently performed.*

CASE 9 • *A 76-year-old patient who underwent bilateral external iliac angioplasty and had a retroperitoneal haemorrhage. He was nursed on the general surgical ward and seen only by a senior house officer following the procedure. Although the patient was deteriorating neither a radiologist nor vascular surgeon were called. The problem was not recognised until the patient had a cardiac arrest and a subsequent postmortem was performed (see also page 19).*

CASE 10 • *An 89-year-old patient suffered a retroperitoneal haematoma following femoral angioplasty performed in a hospital where there was no on-site vascular surgeon (see also page 19).*

CASE 11 • *An 81-year-old patient with claudication, but no rest pain, had an external iliac stent performed. She was considered to be a high risk because of coexisting medical problems. Because of this combination of factors it was the advisors' view that this was an ill-advised procedure.*

Table 1.13: Grade of the most senior doctor who referred the patient	
Grade	Number
Consultant	257
Staff grade	1
SpR Accredited/CCST	6
SpR 4	9
SpR 3	8
SpR 2	4
Visiting SpR	2
SHO 2	1
Other	2
Not known	1
Not answered	12
Total	303

It is reassuring to see that the vast majority (85%) of these patients were referred by a consultant. Of those that were not, the majority were referred by reasonably experienced registrars and in no cases were locums involved.

Radiologist's assessment prior to procedure

Table 1.14: Grade of the most senior radiologist who reviewed the patient before the procedure	
Grade	Number
Consultant	275
SpR Accredited/CCST	5
SpR 4	5
SpR 3	1
Other	2
None	13
Not answered	2
Total	303

The radiologist should not be seen as a technician who performs interventions when requested, but should assess the patient prior to, and after, the procedure and, where necessary, discuss with the referring clinicians. It was encouraging to see that 275/303 (91%) patients were assessed by a consultant radiologist, but disconcerting that there were 13 patients who were not reviewed by a radiologist prior to the procedure (Table 1.14).

Specialty and seniority of radiologist

Key Point

- *The interventional radiologist should have sufficient experience to perform the procedure safely and to deal with any complications that may arise.*

Table 1.15: Specialty of most senior radiologist present	
Specialty	Number
General radiologist with vascular interventional interest	187
Specialist vascular interventional radiologist	101
General radiologist	4
Other	7
Not answered	4
Total	303

In the majority (95%) of cases the most senior radiologist was one with an appropriate special interest in interventional radiology and in only four cases were they designated simply as a 'general radiologist'.

Table 1.16: Grade of most senior doctor performing the procedure	
Grade	Number
Consultant	283
SpR Accredited/CCST	9
SpR 4	6
SpR 3	2
SpR 2	1
Not answered	2
Total	303

Question 1.1: If the most senior operator was not a consultant, was a more senior doctor immediately available?

Yes	12
No	4
Not answered	4
Total	20

The majority of procedures were performed by consultants (93%), with some being performed by registrars indicating that training is in progress (Table 1.16). We do not have the evidence as to whether or not this is sufficient for the future number of consultants required. In 12 of these cases a consultant was immediately available and, whilst this is generally good, in four cases there was no consultant available and this is a situation that should not occur. Some examples of problems which may arise are:

CASE 12 • *A 69-year-old patient with lower limb ischaemia was undergoing an iliac angioplasty and insertion of stent. The radiologist had done only six similar procedures in the previous year. The external iliac artery ruptured during the procedure and attempts to control the bleeding with a balloon failed. There was a delay in getting the patient to theatre (see also page 20).*

CASE 13 • *A 57-year-old patient with alcoholic liver disease and oesophageal varices had a failed TIPS because of inability to puncture the portal vein in a small cirrhotic liver. The radiologist had done only two such cases in the previous three years (see also page 23).*

CASE 14 • *A 67-year-old patient had an attempted renal angioplasty which failed for technical reasons. The radiologist had done only two similar procedures in the last year.*

FACILITIES, PERSONNEL AND MONITORING

Dedicated room

> ### Key Point
>
> • *Interventional vascular radiological procedures should be performed in a dedicated interventional room.*

Table 1.17: Location in which the procedure was performed	
Location	Number
Dedicated interventional room	276
General fluoroscopy room	24
Other	2
Not answered	1
Total	303

In 276 cases the procedure was performed in a dedicated interventional room while in 24 a general fluoroscopy room was used. It is not satisfactory that 8% of procedures were carried out in a general fluoroscopy room; a dedicated interventional room should be available for all cases.

Equipment

> ### Key Points
>
> • *There should be adequate equipment to perform the procedure safely.*
> • *It is the radiologist's responsibility to check the equipment prior to commencing the procedure.*
> • *A designated member of the team should be responsible for 'stock-taking'.*

There were examples where lack of equipment resulted in less than ideal treatment being given:

CASE 15 • *A 77-year-old patient with a tight renal artery stenosis had a renal angioplasty performed. It was thought that a stent should be used, but none was available.*

CASE 16 • *A 54-year-old patient with an occluded femorodistal graft had this cleared with thrombolysis. This unmasked a stenosis for which it was felt a 3 or 4 mm balloon would be ideal. However, there was none available and a 5 mm balloon had to be used. Although, in fact, this did not cause any problem it is not an ideal situation.*

It is essential that all vascular radiology suites are equipped with the full range of stents, angioplasty balloon catheters and other equipment that may be required. There should be a checklist and a designated member of the team responsible for 'stock-taking'. The radiologist performing the procedure has the ultimate responsibility for ensuring that everything which may be needed is present before commencing each procedure.

Shortage of personnel

Key Point

- *There should be sufficient staff to perform the procedure safely.*

Question 1.2: Was there a shortage of personnel in this case?

Yes	4
No	285
Not answered	14
Total	303

If yes, which? (4 cases, answers may be multiple)

Consultant radiologist	1
Radiographer	1
Consultant anaesthetist	1
Nurses	2
Porter	1

Whilst it is encouraging that there was a shortage of personnel in so few cases it is nevertheless vital, if a high standard is to be maintained, to ensure sufficient staff in all cases. The interventional radiology nurse is an important member of the team.

Delays

Key Point

- *There needs to be a sufficient number of fully-staffed interventional radiology sessions for urgent patients to receive their treatment without delay.*

Question 1.3: Were there any delays (between admission and procedure) due to factors other than clinical?

Yes	11
No	285
Not answered	7
Total	303

Table 1.18: Reasons for non-clinical delay between admission and procedure
(11 cases; answers may be multiple)

Reason	Number
Pressure of work	8
Poor communication	2
Shortage of beds	1
Insufficient cover at weekends	1
Vascular radiologist on leave	1
Patient refused	1

Anaesthesia

Question 1.4: Was the procedure performed solely under local anaesthetic or sedation administered by the operator?

Yes	254
No	47
Not answered	2
Total	303

In 254/303 (84%) cases the procedure was performed under local anaesthetic or sedation administered solely by the operator.

An anaesthetist was present for 43 of the procedures and in 30 administered general anaesthesia. In the remainder they were there to administer local anaesthesia and sedation.

Of the 43 anaesthetists, one was an SpR 1, 16 were SpR 3 or higher and twenty were consultants; the grade was not known in the remaining six cases. The X-ray department is a more difficult environment than the operating theatre in which to give an anaesthetic. It is, therefore, inappropriate for an inexperienced anaesthetist to be responsible for such cases.

Monitoring

Key Point

- *Monitoring of pulse oximetry, blood pressure and ECG should be performed during all interventional radiological procedures; this should be done by someone other than the radiologist performing the procedure.*

Table 1.19: Monitoring performed during or immediately after the procedure (303 cases; answers may be multiple)	
Monitoring	Number
Pulse	271
Blood pressure	263
Pulse oximetry	239
ECG	108
Other	30
None	19
Not answered	6

Of concern is the fact that in 19 cases no monitoring was performed, as all patients having interventional procedures should be monitored. In addition, there was no monitoring of the pulse in 32 patients, of the blood pressure in 40 patients, of oxygen saturation in 64 patients and the ECG in 195 patients.

Table 1.20: Responsibility for monitoring the patient's general condition during the procedure (303 cases; answers may be multiple)	
Person	Number
A nurse	211
The operator	97
An anaesthetist	42
Another doctor	17
A radiographer	16
Not answered	1

In 97 cases monitoring was undertaken by the person performing the interventional radiological procedure. In 60 of these monitoring was also being performed by another member of the team. However, in 37 cases the operator was the only person monitoring the patient, and this is a cause for concern. Interventional procedures are frequently technically demanding and it is not possible for the same person to carry these out and adequately monitor the patient. Radiographers are not trained to perform monitoring, and ideally this should be performed by a nurse or an operating department assistant. An oxygen supply should be available and if any sedation in the form of benzodiazepines or opioid drugs is used then the specific antagonists should be available (flumazanil or naloxone respectively)[1]. In all areas where invasive procedures are performed, there should be resuscitation equipment that is regularly checked and core staff trained and regularly updated in resuscitation.

Care following the procedure

Recovery

Question 1.5: Was there a recovery room/area available attached to the procedure suite?

Yes 210
No 88
Not answered 5
Total 303

It is unsatisfactory that in almost one third (29%) of cases there was no recovery area for patients after their interventional procedure. A recovery area should be available.

Intensive and high dependency care

Key Point

- *These patients may be desperately ill and it is essential that ICU/HDU beds are available when required.*

Forty patients were admitted to an intensive care unit (ICU) and 20 to a high dependency unit (HDU) immediately after their procedure, with a further 18 being admitted to ICU and six to HDU after a period on a routine ward. In the remainder admission to ICU/HDU was not felt necessary, except in three cases where the patient's condition did warrant admission to ICU or HDU, but there was no bed available within the hospital in which the procedure took place:

CASE 7 • *A 45-year-old patient with acute on chronic aortoiliac occlusion (see also page 12).*

CASE 17 • *A 44-year-old patient with alcoholic liver disease, together with haematemesis and melaena due to oesophageal varices, was referred for a TIPS procedure. The patient had to be transferred back to the original hospital after the procedure, as there was no HDU bed available. It would have been more satisfactory to keep him at the same hospital.*

CASE 18 • *A 57-year-old patient with acute myeloid leukaemia had a Hickman line inserted for administration of chemotherapy. The procedure was uneventful. A week later he developed coagulase-negative septicaemia. A further week later he became seriously ill despite antibiotics. The Hickman line was removed. There was no ICU or HDU bed available so he was nursed on the general medical ward and died three days later.*

COMPLICATIONS

Table 1.21: Unexpected procedural complications (37 cases; answers may be multiple)	
Complication	Number
Unable to cross the vascular lesion	6
Embolus/thrombosis of run-off vessels	6
Occlusion of artery during procedure	5
Bleeding/haematoma from groin	3
Rupture of iliac artery	3
Thrombosis of brachial artery when used to approach aortoiliac segment	2
Lack of correct-sized balloon	2
Unexpected cardiac arrest during procedure	2
Internal flap in superficial femoral artery	1
Stroke during carotid angioplasty	1
Patient's rest pain so severe he could not lie still	1
Groin puncture site very painful	1
Extravasation of blood from femoropopliteal segment	1
Myocardial infarction during procedure	1
Severe nose bleed during thrombolysis	1
Coagulopathy during embolisation for blood loss	1
Axillary vein thrombosis during SVC stent (cleared at lysis)	1
Tumour more extensive then realised prior to SVC stent	1
Pneumothorax during insertion of Hickman line	1

In 37 cases there were unanticipated procedural complications; in three of these there were two unexpected complications.

The list of complications in Table 1.21 is typical of those that arise during interventional procedures. The vast majority were unavoidable and dealt with appropriately. There were particular problems in a few cases which are discussed later.

Table 1.22: Postprocedural complications	
(303 cases; answers may be multiple)	
Complication	**Number**
Respiratory distress	46
Low cardiac output/other cardiac problems	45
Renal failure	44
Peripheral ischaemia	34
Haemorrhage/postoperative bleeding requiring transfusion or surgical endovascular intervention	31
Cardiac arrest	29
Hepatic failure	25
Generalised sepsis	22
Stroke or other neurological problems	15
Other organ failure	11
Persistent coma	9
Pulmonary embolus	8
Problem with analgesia	6
Nutritional problems	6
Pressure sores	3
Wound infection/dehiscence	1
Endocrine system failure	1
DVT	1
Urinary retention/catheter blockage	1
Other	29
Not answered	110
None	20

With the exception of haemorrhage and postoperative bleeding, which were more common in patients having thrombolysis, there was no obvious correlation between any particular procedures and subsequent complications.

Specific problems

Level of puncture

Key Point

- *Cannulation of the femoral artery should always be below the inguinal ligament to avoid the danger of retroperitoneal haematoma. Medical and nursing staff must be aware of the risks of this serious complication in order to act early when necessary.*

There were several cases where retroperitoneal bleeding occurred:

CASE 9 • *A 76-year-old patient who underwent bilateral external iliac angioplasty and had a retroperitoneal haemorrhage (see also page 13).*

CASE 10 • *An 89-year-old patient had a high femoral puncture in order to perform a superficial femoral artery angioplasty. She developed a massive retroperitoneal haematoma. There was no on-site vascular surgeon on the day of the angioplasty (see also page 13).*

CASE 19 • *An 83-year-old patient with an acutely ischaemic left leg, due to a left external iliac thrombosis, had thrombolysis followed by balloon angioplasty. Four days later he died and at postmortem was found to have a retroperitoneal haematoma.*

Great care must always be taken to keep the level of puncture below the inguinal ligament so that bleeding is recognised immediately. Above the inguinal ligament a very large amount of blood may be lost in the retroperitoneal space and may not be recognised until the patient is clinically in the advanced stages of shock. Elderly patients with heart disease make up quite a high proportion of patients having angioplasties and they do not tolerate blood loss well. If the radiologist or any other clinician is at all suspicious, an ultrasound or CT scan should be performed to confirm and perhaps monitor the amount of bleeding. It is also essential to warn clinical staff looking after the patient and ensure they are aware of the possibility and dangers of retroperitoneal bleeding. The patient should be nursed on a specialist vascular ward where nurses and medical staff are fully aware of the risk of the possibility of development of retroperitoneal haematoma and its serious consequences. If bleeding does not stop the patient must be taken to theatre to suture the bleeding point before it is too late.

Lower limb revascularisation

Key Points

- *The interventional radiologist should have sufficient experience, facilities and equipment to perform the procedure safely and to deal with any complications that may arise.*
- *It should always be possible to control bleeding of a ruptured iliac artery either temporarily with a balloon catheter or permanently with a covered stent.*
- *A 'rupture box' containing all necessary equipment should be available in every interventional radiology department.*

If angioplasties and stents performed in the iliac, femoral and popliteal arteries are included then a total of 11 692 of these procedures were performed, of whom 101 patients died, giving a mortality of less than 1% (0.9%) (Table 1.6, page 8). Bearing in mind that a significant number of these patients are severe arteriopaths with critical ischaemia, on whom vascular surgeons are not keen to operate, then these results are generally very creditable. However, there was some cause for concern in three cases where the external iliac artery was ruptured during angioplasty.

CASE 12 • *A 69-year-old patient had an iliac angioplasty and stent. The artery ruptured, the bleeding was controlled with a balloon, but because of ischaemia was let down again before the patient was taken to theatre! There was a delay of forty minutes in getting the patient to theatre (see also page 14).*

CASE 20 • *A 74-year-old patient had an external iliac angioplasty which ruptured the artery. No radiological measures were taken to try and control the bleeding. The patient was taken to theatre urgently for iliofemoral bypass.*

CASE 21 • *A 63-year-old patient having an iliac stent placed had a rupture of the iliac artery with the stent in situ. A covered stent would almost certainly have stopped the bleeding.*

These cases illustrate the need for suitable experience and ability of the operator and the availability of equipment. It should be possible to control the bleeding of a ruptured iliac artery permanently with a covered stent and these are commercially available. If this does not control the bleeding then a balloon should give temporary control until the patient can be taken to theatre, which obviously needs to be done as a matter of great urgency. It is recommended that every interventional radiology department should have a 'rupture box' containing all the necessary equipment, which can be opened at a moment's notice, to deal with this emergency.

The conclusion, therefore, is that angioplasty should not be performed unless the radiologist has the experience to recognise, and ability and equipment to deal with, complications. The immediate help of a vascular surgical team should be available when needed.

Thrombolysis

Key Points

- *There is a danger of cerebral haemorrhage with thrombolytic therapy particularly when used in the elderly (over 75 years) or if too large a dose is given.*

- *Patients having continued thrombolytic therapy after leaving the vascular radiology suite should be nursed on an HDU or specialist vascular ward where there are an adequate number of nurses to monitor them closely.*

Thrombolysis can be extremely useful in dissolving clot that has formed in the blood vessel or graft, but it must be remembered that at best it can merely restore the vessel to the state it was in prior to the thrombus forming. The underlying cause will still need to be treated, for example an arterial thrombosis secondary to a stenosis will need an angioplasty once the thrombus has been cleared. Similarly, in a peripheral arterial embolus, or a deep vein thrombosis, anticoagulation will be needed to prevent further thrombosis. There is a risk of bleeding both locally and at distance, which may include spontaneous retroperitoneal haemorrhage or, more seriously, cerebral haemorrhage. The incidence of minor haemorrhage is about 15%, major haemorrhage about 5%[2] and haemorrhagic stroke is 1%. Other studies have found the risk of stroke (both haemorrhagic and ischaemic) to be 2.3%[3]. The risks seem to be greater in patients over 75 years[4]. Although patients with simple emboli and normal peripheral arteries are a rarity, nevertheless where the clinical features strongly suggest an embolus then surgery may give better results, especially in the elderly[5]. The risk of bleeding increases with a larger dose and a longer period of administration. The question of dose has been discussed in detail[5], but absolute recommendations on drugs and dosage are not possible on available data, although current practice has moved away from the use of streptokinase to rt-PA.

Some examples of problems with thrombolysis include:

CASE 22 • *An 87-year-old patient was given thrombolysis for a thrombosed femoropopliteal graft and died due to cerebral haemorrhage.*

CASE 23 • *An 83-year-old patient having thrombolysis for a thrombosed iliac artery died of cerebral haemorrhage.*

There were three other patients aged 84, 87 and 97 years who, although they did not suffer a cerebral haemorrhage, were considered by the advisors to be too old to have treatment by thrombolysis.

There were two further patients in whom it was felt the dose was inappropriate:

CASE 24 • *A 77-year-old patient had an ischaemic left arm due to subclavian thrombosis. This was treated with streptokinase 20 000 units per hour and heparin 15 000 units per hour. This was continued for 18 hours when a check angiogram showed only partial thrombolysis. The patient subsequently died of angina and a stroke. No postmortem was performed and therefore it is unknown whether this was a haemorrhagic or thrombotic stroke, but either way the advisors considered that this was too large a dose of streptokinase.*

CASE 25 • *A 68-year-old patient had thrombolysis for an acute occlusion of the right superficial femoral artery due to an underlying popliteal aneurysm. He was given 50 mg of rt-PA in 5 mg aliquots over a two hour period. One hour later the patient was taken to theatre for a femorodistal bypass. As far as was possible to ascertain from the questionnaire the surgeon was not aware of how large a dose had been given. Certainly the advisors considered that this was too great a dose. The patient died 24 hours later and although postmortem did show some haemorrhage around both puncture sites death was due to peripheral vascular disease.*

Although thrombolysis can be very effective, its use does carry significant risks particularly in patients over 75 years, and even more so over the age of 80. However, one needs to bear in mind that surgery for acute ischaemia in elderly patients is also hazardous with a mortality rate of about 30%[6]. Whatever choice of treatment is given it is essential that the patient is warned of the risks of both thrombolysis and surgery, and indeed of not undergoing either. Certainly the risks with thrombolysis are greater the higher the dose used and the longer it is given. Although it is not possible to give absolute guidelines, since there is insufficient data, the advisors considered that the normal dose of streptokinase for continuous infusion should not exceed 5000 units per hour, but that it is probably better to use rt-PA with the dose not normally exceeding 0.5-1.0 mg per hour, although it may be greater if the pulse spray infusion is used[7].

Patients having thrombolysis need close observation for early detection of any complications and for monitoring the response, so that it is given for the shortest possible time, but also so that an adequate amount has been given to clear the vessel. Therefore they should go to an HDU or specialist vascular ward with an adequate number of nurses to monitor closely, and the easy facility for repeat angiograms as required. Case 7 (see pages 12 and 18) was an example where the advisors thought it would have been preferable to manage the patient on an HDU or ICU. The view of the advisors was that wherever there is ongoing thrombolysis the patient should be nursed on an HDU or a specialist vascular ward.

Embolisation

Key Points

- *If embolisation is to be used for severe persistent bleeding, radiologists should be called sooner rather than later in order to instigate treatment before a serious coagulopathy has developed.*
- *It must be remembered that embolisation to stop bleeding can occasionally cause ischaemic infarction.*

Table 1.6 (page 8) showed that embolisation was used via the internal iliac artery for uterine fibroids, for the treatment of bleeding pelvic fractures, for renal disease, most commonly to reduce the vascularity prior to removing a large tumour, and for gastrointestinal bleeding. Other sites of embolisation included the liver for treatment of secondaries, particularly for carcinoid tumour or AV malformations, and embolisation of the internal mammary artery for haemoptysis due to lung cancer.

When embolisation is used for persistent bleeding, early communication with the vascular radiologist is necessary if embolisation is going to have a chance to be effective before a serious coagulopathy has developed (see case 3 and case 4 on page 12).

Gastrointestinal bleeding can be particularly problematic both to diagnose where the bleeding is coming from and to treat adequately. Embolisation can be extremely useful, but the following illustrate the problems that can occur:

CASE 26 • *A 78-year-old patient with severe colonic bleeding was treated with selective Sterispon embolisation which successfully stopped the bleeding. The radiologist wrote in the notes: ' There is a risk of colonic infarction following this procedure and the patient should be closely observed for signs of this.' Colonic infarction did indeed develop and the patient required a laparotomy to remove ischaemic bowel on the following day.*

CASE 27 • *A 74-year-old patient with persistent bleeding from a duodenal ulcer was treated with coil embolisation of the pancreatoduodenal arteries. This controlled the bleeding, but 13 days later the duodenum perforated and it was thought that ischaemia had played a part in this.*

CASE 28 • *A 67-year-old patient had a Whipples operation which was complicated by a pancreatic leak, sepsis and a subsequent false aneurysm of the hepatic artery which bled. This was treated by coil embolisation controlling the bleeding. The patient died a few days later of multiple organ failure which was thought to be due to sepsis, although in fact postmortem examination showed hepatic necrosis.*

CASE 29 • *A 51-year-old patient had embolisation for bleeding uterine fibroids. The ischaemic uterus became infected and the patient subsequently died.*

While embolisation is an extremely useful therapeutic measure[8] it must be remembered that it can cut off the blood supply to the affected area sufficiently to cause ischaemic necrosis. It is important to be aware of this possibility and recognise and treat it early if it should occur.

SVC stent

Two hundred and sixty-six of these were performed and seventeen of the patients died (6%). These procedures are performed for advanced malignancy which has obstructed the superior vena cava causing venous engorgement of the upper half of the body. In all these cases it was thought that death was due to the underlying disease, and that SVC stenting is a useful therapeutic measure[9].

Central venous access

Over 3000 of these were performed, for haemodialysis, the administration of chemotherapy for malignancy or for long-term intravenous feeding. Of the 36 patients who died, one had a pneumothorax, which was felt to have contributed to the patient's death. In all the remainder it was considered that death was due to the underlying disease. Thus, this is a very safe procedure in the hands of a radiologist.

Transjugular intrahepatic portosystemic shunt (TIPS)

Acute variceal bleeding which fails to respond to medical management remains the primary indication for TIPS and accounts for over 80% of cases performed. Most of these patients are desperately ill and operating on them is almost always more hazardous[10,11]. Of the 158 cases performed, 27 patients died (17%). Bearing in mind the very serious nature of the disease these were felt to be acceptable results. It has, however, been suggested that centres undertaking less than five cases per year are unlikely to achieve the required expertise[11]; this does argue for referral of patients to centres with a large experience of these procedures. Case 13 (see page 14) reinforces this point.

DVT prophylaxis

Question 1.6: Were any measures taken (before, during or after the procedure) to prevent venous thromboembolism?

Yes 115
No 169
Not answered 18
Not known 1
Total 303

Bearing in mind that most of these patients were middle-aged or elderly, with a significant number of other medical problems, and the majority of them generally unfit as judged by the ASA grade, according to the THRIFT[12] they should probably all have had some form of DVT prophylaxis, mainly subcutaneous heparin. However, the advisors were not unanimous on this, particularly bearing in mind that many diagnostic angiograms are performed as day cases.

POSTMORTEM EXAMINATIONS

Key Point

- *In one in eight of the postmortems performed the pathological finding was different from that expected by the clinical team. This surely must have educational benefit and is the reason why more postmortems should be performed.*

Ninety-six of the 303 deaths were reported to the coroner and of these 58 had a coroner's postmortem performed. Of the remaining 245 cases, only 15 patients had a hospital postmortem. Of the 73 postmortems performed, in only seven did a radiologist attend and in only four did another clinician do so. A copy of the postmortem report was only received by the team in 37/73 (51%) cases.

Question 1.7: Did the pathological information confirm the team's clinical impression?

Yes	56
No	8
None received	2
Not answered	6
Not known	1
Total	73

In eight out of the 64 cases on which this information was available, the pathological finding at postmortem was different from that which the clinical team was expecting. The details are as follows:

CASE 28 • *A 67-year-old patient had embolisation to control bleeding from the hepatic artery. Postmortem showed unsuspected hepatic necrosis (see also page 22).*

CASE 30 • *A 60-year-old patient had embolisation for hepatic metastases. He was thought to have died as a result of this but postmortem showed death was due to an unsuspected haemorrhage into a cerebral metastasis.*

CASE 31 • *A 60-year-old patient was thought to have carcinoma of the colon and heart failure. At postmortem she was found to have ischaemic colitis and death was due to a pulmonary embolism caused by a DVT.*

CASE 32 • *A 69-year-old patient was admitted with a femoral vein thrombosis. She was treated with heparin which had to be stopped when she had a gastrointestinal bleed. An IVC filter was inserted. She was thought to have died from gastrointestinal bleeding but at postmortem no source could be found. There was a DVT of the left leg and an old pulmonary embolus, but death was caused by acute myocardial ischaemia due to coronary artery atheroma with plaque rupture.*

CASE 33 • *A 76-year-old patient had a stent for renal artery stenosis. Despite having heparin prophylaxis he was thought to have died from pulmonary embolism. Postmortem showed no evidence of an embolus, and death was due to congestive cardiac failure due to myocardial infarction.*

CASE 34 • *A 67-year-old patient had a stent and thrombolysis for SVC thrombosis secondary to enlarged mediastinal lymph nodes thought to be due to a bronchogenic carcinoma or possibly a lymphoma. Postmortem showed no evidence of either but death was due to metastases of intestinal origin.*

CASE 35 • *A 63-year-old patient had a stent for SVC obstruction due to mediastinal lymphadenopathy. He was given dexamethasone. Two days later he died of circulatory collapse. Postmortem showed death was due to peritonitis caused by a completely unsuspected perforated duodenal ulcer.*

CASE 36 • *An 87-year-old patient had a popliteal angioplasty for a critically ischaemic leg. Death was thought to be due to sepsis from the ischaemic limb, but postmortem showed it was caused by peritonitis due to a perforated duodenal ulcer.*

These cases illustrate why postmortem examinations need to be performed more frequently.

AUDIT AND AVAILABILITY OF PATIENT RECORDS

Key Point

- *It is as important for radiologists to assess and audit their results as it is for other clinical staff.*

It is disappointing that in only 125/303 (41%) cases was the patient's death discussed at a local audit or quality control meeting. The figure should be very much higher. The need for radiologists to assess and audit their results is every bit as important as it is for other clinical staff.

It was also disappointing that in 82/303 (27%) cases there was difficulty in obtaining the patient's notes and in 64 cases (21%) either notes or images were unavailable. The most common problem was finding the death certificate (43 cases) and other problems included obtaining a postmortem report (14 cases), postprocedure notes (12 cases) and the images (10 cases). With the introduction of clinical governance it is to be hoped that the systems will be in place for all notes and other information to be readily available.

Vascular Radiology

NATIONAL CEPOD 25

2 INTERVENTIONAL NEUROVASCULAR RADIOLOGY

RECOMMENDATIONS

- The number of neuroradiologists and support staff needs to increase to ensure a satisfactory on-call rota, including weekends (page 36).

- There is a need for recognised training programmes in neuroradiology to meet the demand for more consultants (page 36).

- Monitoring of the patient should be performed in all cases, and should be the responsibility of someone other than the neuroradiologist performing the procedure (page 38).

- It is important that there are sufficient facilities for a prompt emergency service, and ICU/HDU beds for subsequent care (pages 36, 39).

2. INTERVENTIONAL NEUROVASCULAR RADIOLOGY

INTRODUCTION

Key Points

- *In all cases the procedures were performed by appropriately experienced specialists and there was a high standard of care.*

- *By far the most common condition was subarachnoid haemorrhage due to intracranial aneurysm, treated by detachable coils.*

- *Use of these techniques has developed from almost none in 1992, to over 800 patients a year, with very little increase in staff or facilities.*

- *The majority of patients are otherwise medically fit with good long-term outlook after successful treatment.*

- *Patients who survive an initial subarachnoid haemorrhage have an increasing risk of a further bleed as each day passes; treatment is therefore a matter of urgency.*

This is an important study, being the first time an audit of deaths has been carried out for this specialty.

Over the past two decades or more, interventional neurovascular radiology has become an important and sophisticated specialty in its own right. It has benefited from the same advances in technology as coronary angioplasty and peripheral vascular interventional radiology. The specialty has developed with the close cooperation of neurosurgeons and neurologists and requires the full neuroscience support team, including other disciplines. In particular, access to high dependency and intensive care units is needed every bit as much as these facilities are required after neurosurgery.

The most common problem is the prevention of further bleeding from subarachnoid haemorrhage (SAH) in patients with intracranial aneurysms. Arteriovenous malformations (AVMs) of the brain are a less common cause of cerebral haemorrhage. These conditions are treated by embolisation which may be by the use of detachable coils for aneurysms, or the tissue adhesive N butyl cyanoacrylate (Histoacryl or NBCA), or newer liquid embolic agents which are just becoming available, for AVMs. The liquid agents such as cyanoacrylates have the advantage that they permeate into very small vessels and reach far distally, thus enabling occlusion of the nidus of the malformation on a permanent basis. A number of ingenious devices have been invented which enable, for example, the coils to stay attached until they are in precisely the correct position and then released. The most notable is the Guglielmi detachable platinum microcoil (GDC) which is

soldered at the end of an insulated stainless-steel guidewire and is detached by passing a current through it which causes electrolysis of the exposed detachment zone[13,14].

The method of embolisation that is used depends on the precise detail of the vasculature to be embolised and the amount of risk there is to the surrounding normal tissue. Embolisation may also be used for cerebral tumours.

Vasospasm of the cerebral vessels occurs in about 20% of patients following aneurysmal haemorrhage. Treatment for this may take the form of either super-selective injection of papaverine or of angioplasty to the cerebral vessel in spasm, or a combination of both.

Cerebrovascular occlusive disease may be treated by angioplasty, or angioplasty and stent, and thrombotic disease may be treated by thrombolysis.

When thrombolysis is used for cerebral vascular thrombosis, it runs all the same risks as it does elsewhere of causing haemorrhage both locally where it is applied and at a distance. It is particularly likely to cause a problem if used for thromboembolic complications following treatment for SAH due to intracranial aneurysm and should be used with great caution, particularly under these circumstances.

DATA COLLECTION

Data was requested from all NHS hospitals undertaking these procedures in England, Scotland, Wales and Northern Ireland. Participation was voluntary and some hospitals chose, for a variety of reasons, not to participate.

Information on the total number of patients undergoing interventional neurovascular radiology procedures on a monthly basis, together with notification of any deaths occurring within 30 days of the procedure, were collected for the period 1 April 1998 - 31 March 1999.

GENERAL DATA ANALYSIS

Monthly returns of procedures performed

27 hospitals agreed to participate in the study. Each hospital was required to send in a monthly return of all patients undergoing interventional neurovascular radiological procedures in the hospital. A total of 324 forms should therefore have been received. The return rate of monthly data is shown in Figure 2.1.

A regional breakdown of the number of monthly forms received is given in Table 2.1. The return rate of monthly forms was excellent; only North Thames (75%) and North West (89%) failed to achieve complete returns.

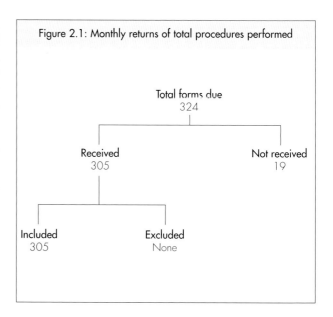

Figure 2.1: Monthly returns of total procedures performed

Table 2.1: Monthly returns by region				
Region	Number of participating hospitals	Monthly forms received	Monthly forms expected	Return rate
Anglia & Oxford	2	24	24	100%
North Thames	6	54	72	75%
North West	3	32	36	89%
Northern & Yorkshire	4	48	48	100%
South & West	2	24	24	100%
South Thames	3	36	36	100%
Trent	2	24	24	100%
West Midlands	1	12	12	100%
Wales	1	12	12	100%
Northern Ireland	1	12	12	100%
Scotland	2	24	24	100%

Reported deaths

Figure 2.2 shows that a total of 41 reports of deaths within 30 days of a procedure were received. Of these, two were excluded from further analysis: one was received after the deadline of 31 August 1999 and one remained incomplete despite all efforts to identify missing information.

A regional breakdown of the 39 included deaths is shown in Table 2.2.

The differences in numbers of deaths reported by each region reflects the total number of procedures undertaken, together with the completeness of the data submitted.

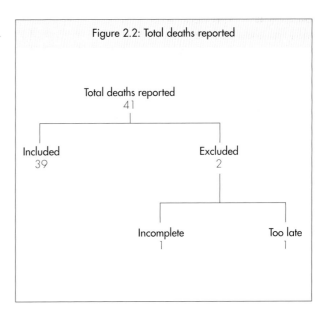

Figure 2.2: Total deaths reported

Table 2.2: Deaths reported to NCEPOD by region	
Region	Deaths reported
Anglia & Oxford	8
North Thames	0
North West	6
Northern & Yorkshire	7
South & West	2
South Thames	4
Trent	4
West Midlands	1
Wales	1
Northern Ireland	2
Scotland	4
Total	39

Distribution of deaths

Key Points

- *The majority of patients who died did so within a week of the procedure as a direct result of subarachnoid haemorrhage.*
- *The peak age groups were between 30 and 60 years with equal sex distribution.*

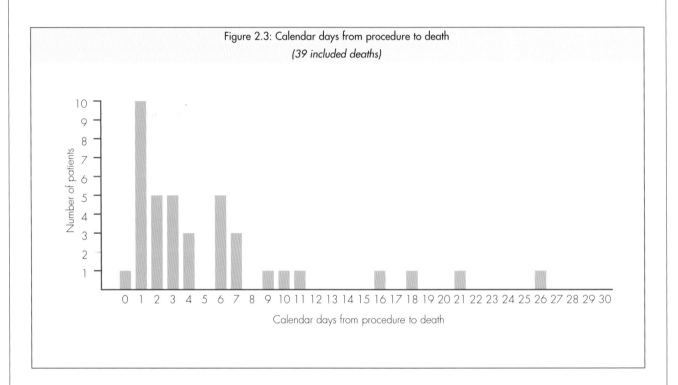

Figure 2.3: Calendar days from procedure to death
(39 included deaths)

Figure 2.3 shows the distribution of the number of calendar days between procedure (day 0) and death. It is interesting to note that the majority of deaths occurred in the first few days following neurovascular procedures and there are very few deaths after more than a week. This is in contrast to Figure 1.3 on page 6 showing the distribution of deaths following interventional vascular radiological procedures where there is a wider spread over the month following the procedure. This is presumably because neurovascular patients die as a result of their intracranial haemorrhage, whereas the interventional vascular patients die as a result of their coexisting medical conditions.

It is interesting to note from Figure 2.4 how much younger these patients are on average than those having interventional vascular radiology (see Figure 1.4 on page 6). The vascular patients also have an obvious preponderance of males whereas there is no such difference in the neurovascular patients.

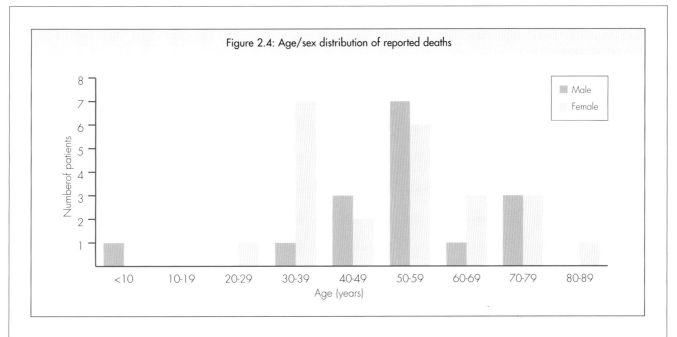

Figure 2.4: Age/sex distribution of reported deaths

Number of patients (y-axis, 1–8)
Age (years) (x-axis): <10, 10-19, 20-29, 30-39, 40-49, 50-59, 60-69, 70-79, 80-89

Legend: Male, Female

Distribution, return and analysis of questionnaires

Questionnaires were sent to the consultant radiologist responsible for the care of each of the 39 patients included. Figure 2.5 shows the return and analysis rates of questionnaires sent.

The return rate of 92% was excellent; in two cases the radiologist indicated that he/she was too busy to complete the questionnaire and the third gave no reason for failing to return the form. It was not necessary to exclude any questionnaires from subsequent analysis.

Table 2.3 shows the returns by region and the majority achieved a 100% return rate; indeed the overall return rate of 92% was due to a nil return rate from South & West and West Midlands.

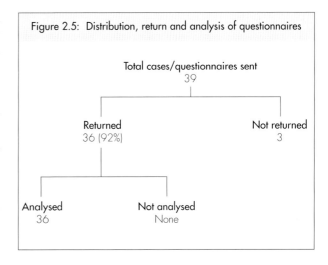

Figure 2.5: Distribution, return and analysis of questionnaires

Total cases/questionnaires sent
39

Returned 36 (92%) — Not returned 3

Analysed 36 — Not analysed None

Table 2.3: Regional distribution and return rates			
Region	Questionnaires distributed	Questionnaires returned	Return rate
Anglia & Oxford	8	8	100%
North Thames	0	0	-
North West	6	6	100%
Northern & Yorkshire	7	7	100%
South & West	2	0	-
South Thames	4	4	100%
Trent	4	4	100%
West Midlands	1	0	-
Wales	1	1	100%
Northern Ireland	2	2	100%
Scotland	4	4	100%
Total	39	36	92%

Procedures

Key Points

- *By far the most common condition was subarachnoid haemorrhage due to intracranial aneurysm treated by detachable coils.*
- *A mortality rate of approximately 3% for detachable coil treatment is low considering the very serious nature of the disease.*

Table 2.4 Neurovascular interventions			Total performed	Deaths	
Condition	**Procedure**		**Total performed**	**Deaths**	
Aneurysm	Endosaccular occlusion	GDC	802	25	(3%)
		Other coils	7		
	Parent vessel occlusion		75	5	(7%)
	Spasm	Papaverine	24		-
		Angioplasty	0		-
		Papaverine + angioplasty	1		-
	Thrombolysis		7		-
Arteriovenous malformation (AVM)	Brain	Pial AVM	293		
		Dural AVM	40		-
		CC fistula	30	1	(3%)
		Vein of Galen malformation	21		-
		Other	12		-
	Craniofacial		23		-
	Spine	Dural	28		-
		Other	16		-
Tumour	Brain		84		-
	Head & neck		42		-
	Spine		20		-
Cerebrovascular disease	Occlusive disease	Angioplasty + stent	32	2	(6%)
	Thrombotic disease	Arterial thrombolysis	10	2	(20%)
		Venous thrombolysis	3	1	(33%)
Other			46		-
Total			**1616**	**36**	**(2%)**

Table 2.4 shows that by far the greatest number of procedures performed, and subsequent deaths, were for occlusion of aneurysms. It should be noted that AVMs usually require several treatments over a period of months, therefore exaggerating their numbers, whereas aneurysms are usually only treated once. The overall mortality rate is low for a serious disease where the clinical grade of the patient is a major factor in the outcome.

PATIENT PROFILE

The report hereafter deals only with those patients who died.

Urgency of procedure

Key Points

- *Patients who survive a subarachnoid haemorrhage have a 4% risk of a further bleed in the first 24 hours and a 1% risk per day thereafter.*
- *The majority of patients were treated as emergency or urgent cases.*
- *Detachable coils were introduced to the UK in 1992 and their use has risen from none to over 800 patients treated in a year.*

Following a subarachnoid haemorrhage the likelihood of a further bleed is 4% in the first 24 hours and thereafter 1% per day[15]. It is, therefore, very important that patients are treated urgently.

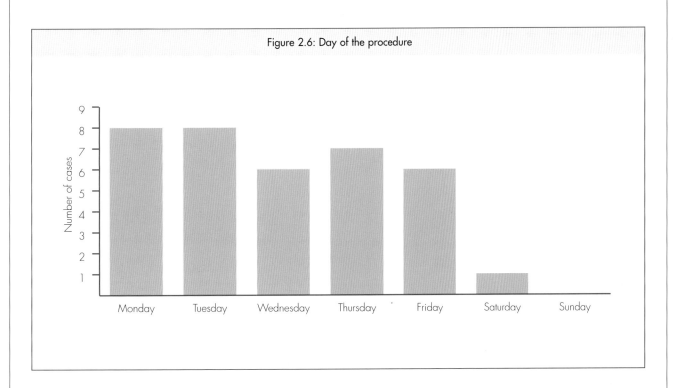

Figure 2.6: Day of the procedure

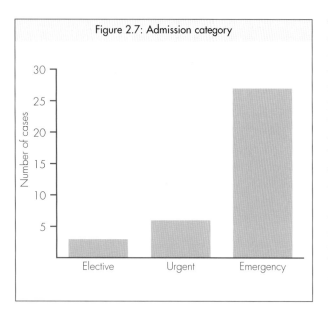

Figure 2.7: Admission category

Thirty of the patients were admitted as an inpatient from another acute hospital or directly from the A&E department, and the majority were admitted to a neurosurgery ward, ICU or HDU under the care of a neurosurgeon. In no patient was there thought to be a deterioration in their condition during transfer, but in two patients there was a delay in referral or admission, though details are lacking. In a further two patients there were delays between admission and procedure, due to factors other than clinical ones:

CASE 1 • *A 59-year-old patient with a subarachnoid haemorrhage was delayed three days for GDC embolisation of her aneurysm due to the heavy workload caused by other patients. The patient died from rupture of the aneurysm during the procedure. This is a recognised complication of this procedure and not related to the delay.*

CASE 2 • *A 56-year-old patient with a subarachnoid haemorrhage was delayed due to a shortage of anaesthetic and nursing staff at the weekend. Death was due to rebleed because of incomplete coil occlusion, and therefore not caused by the delay.*

There has been an enormous increase in the workload of interventional neuroradiologists over the last ten years, mainly due to the introduction of the Guglielmi detachable coil (GDC). Their use has risen from none prior to 1992, when they were first marketed in the UK, to over 800 in the last year, and yet there has been very little increase in the number of neuroradiologists or support staff. Most of this work is urgent or emergency and there is some evidence from this study that this is having an adverse effect on the service provided, particularly in relation to weekend work. The advisors considered that this is a very real problem and considerably greater than the evidence in this report would suggest. A possible short-term solution would be sharing emergency cover, particularly at weekends, with neighbouring units. In many places this is not possible for geographical reasons. The only satisfactory long-term solution is for a steady and progressive increase in staff, which will take time due to training implications for neuroradiologists and support staff. There is a need for recognised training programmes in neuroradiology to be set up in order to meet the consultant expansion which is needed.

Fitness of the patient

Key Points

- *Comorbidities are relatively low when compared with vascular radiology or general surgical patients and probably represent those in the general population of equivalent age.*
- *The prognosis depends on the neurological grading based on the Glasgow Coma Scale (GCS) rather than the ASA grade.*

The majority of neurovascular patients were generally fairly fit when compared with, for example, the large number of comorbidities found in the interventional vascular radiology group (see Table 1.9, page 11) or many general surgical patients[16].

Coexisting problems (other than the main diagnosis) existed in 14/36 (39%) patients and these are shown in Table 2.5.

Table 2.5: Coexisting medical problems (14 cases; answers may be multiple)	
Coexisting medical problem	Number
Respiratory	8
Cardiac	4
Vascular	4
Musculoskeletal	2
Psychiatric	2
Sepsis	2
Alcohol-related problems	1
Diabetes mellitus	1
Malignancy	1
Neurological	1
Renal	1

Figure 2.8 shows the ASA status of the patients; details of assessment of ASA status are given on page 11.

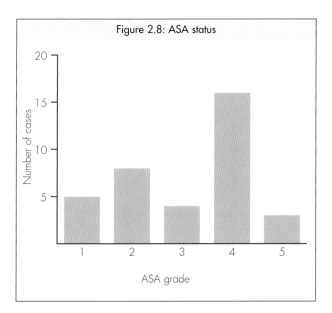

Figure 2.8: ASA status

Thirteen patients (36%) were graded 1 or 2 and most of those in ASA grades 4 and 5 were so graded because of a poor level of consciousness rather than because of cardiovascular or respiratory problems. Although assessed routinely by anaesthetists the ASA grade is not normally used by neuroradiologists, who are far more concerned with the level of consciousness as measured by the Glasgow Coma Scale (GCS).

Table 2.6 shows the World Federation of Neurological Surgeons (WFNS) grading scale that is used following SAH; it is based on the Glasgow Coma Scale.

Table 2.6: Modified Glasgow Coma Scale (GCS)		
GCS	WFNS grade	Number
GCS 15	Grade 1	14
GCS 14-13	Grade 2	9
GCS 14-13+motor deficit	Grade 3	3
GCS 12-7	Grade 4	4
GCS 6-3	Grade 5	6
Total		36

This classification is a useful prognostic indicator as the first two have a good prognosis, with a procedure related mortality of 5-10%, whereas the lower three have a poor prognosis with a mortality of 40-50% following treatment. Without treatment the overall mortality at six months is 50%[17].

The outlook for patients undergoing neuroradiological intervention depends on their GCS rather than their previous medical condition. Prior to their SAH most of the patients are as fit and well as the general population, and following successful treatment return to a near-normal life expectancy. This makes it particularly important that the facilities for their treatment are as good as it is possible to be.

FACILITIES, PERSONNEL AND MONITORING

Key Point

- *All procedures were performed by appropriately experienced specialists in a dedicated interventional room.*

Seniority and specialty of the radiologist

Thirty-five out of the 36 cases were performed by a consultant and one by a specialist registrar with a CCST, with a consultant present.

Table 2.7: Specialty of the most senior radiologist present	
Specialty	Number
Specialist neuroradiologist	33
Specialist interventional vascular radiologist	1
Neurosurgeon with training in radiology	1
Not stated	1
Total	36

Table 2.7 shows that in all cases there was an appropriately experienced specialist present.

Dedicated room

All cases were performed in a dedicated interventional room.

Monitoring

All patients had monitoring of their pulse, blood pressure and pulse oximetry; 34 had ECG monitoring. Thirty-one patients had a general anaesthetic, three received local anaesthetic with sedation and two had local anaesthetic alone, administered by the radiologist. In all 34 cases where an anaesthetist was present they monitored the patient. Of the two cases performed under local anaesthetic, in one the monitoring was done by a nurse and in the other by the neuroradiologist performing the procedure. The latter is unacceptable as monitoring should be performed by a member of the team who is not preoccupied with what may be the very demanding technicalities of the procedure.

Anaesthesia

Thirty-one out of the 36 procedures were performed under general anaesthetic and three under sedation administered by an anaesthetist. In 27 of these 34 cases, the anaesthetist was a consultant and in a further four the anaesthetist was an accredited specialist registrar. In two cases the anaesthetist was an SpR 4 and in one an SpR 3. Thus in all cases the anaesthetist was appropriately experienced.

Question 2.1: Was there non-medical help with anaesthesia?

Yes	30
No	5
Not answered	1
Total	36

If yes, who (30 cases; answers may be multiple)

Radiographer	1
Trained anaesthetic nurse	9
Trained operating department assistant	13
Operating department orderly	7
Other	1

In five cases the anaesthetist did not have a trained assistant; one should be available for all patients having a general anaesthetic. This is particularly important in the X-ray department being a more difficult environment than the operating theatre and distant from other immediate anaesthetic assistance.

Care following the procedure

Intensive and high dependency care

> ## Key Point
>
> - *It is essential that ICU/HDU beds are available for neurovascular radiological patients, in whom there is an ever-present danger of the development of serious complications.*

Twenty-one patients were admitted to an intensive care unit (ICU) and nine to a high dependency unit (HDU) immediately after their procedure, with a further four being admitted to ICU after a period on the ward. One patient, a child of 18 months, was transferred to another hospital which had a paediatric intensive care unit, and a further case was managed on a neurosurgical ward:

CASE 3 • *A 71-year-old patient had a subarachnoid haemorrhage treated by GDCs and developed severe vasospasm. There was no ICU or HDU bed available and he had to be transferred back to the neurosurgical ward.*

Vasospasm is a very serious condition which may require a combination of hypervolaemia, hypertension and haemodilution (Triple H therapy). Only on an HDU can this be done adequately or, if the patient needs ventilation, an ICU bed is required.

It is essential that ICU/HDU beds are available for the postprocedure care of these patients in whom there is an ever-present danger of serious complications occurring and, therefore, a need for specialist intensive care.

COMPLICATIONS

Table 2.8: Postprocedural complications (36 cases; answers may be multiple)	
Complication	Number
Cerebral oedema	10
Haemorrhage from aneurysm	8
Thromboembolic event (CNS)	8
Persistent coma	6
Respiratory distress	5
Haemorrhage from other causes	3
Migration of coils or other embolic agents	3
Hydrocephalus	2
Low cardiac output/other cardiac problems	2
Other organ failure	2
Generalised sepsis	1
Other	8
Not answered	2
None	1

Many of the complications shown in Table 2.8 are, or may be, related to the initial pathology, e.g. hydrocephalus, cerebral oedema or persistent coma. The main problems were CNS thromboembolic events and haemorrhage from an aneurysm, both of which may result in brain oedema and persistent coma, the other two common complications listed. Systemic heparin is normally given to prevent these CNS thromboembolic events, and in 32 patients this was monitored using the Activated Clotting Time (ACT), while in two heparin was given with no monitoring. In addition, three had aspirin, one had another antiplatelet agent and only two had no treatment aimed at preventing thromboembolic problems. Several patients were given thrombolysis following a thromboembolic complication and then subsequently had a further fatal rebleed.

The advisors' view was that patients should normally be given systemic anticoagulation (heparin) during these procedures, and that the dose should be monitored using the ACT. Patients who have bled from an intracranial aneurysm should not normally be given thrombolysis, even if they do develop CNS thromboembolic complications, because of the risk of a further bleed although, at present, there is insufficient data to rule out this mode of treatment completely. It was also thought by the advisors that specific antiplatelet therapy should be given, although there is no systematic data to support either this or the monitoring with ACT.

Of those complications described as 'other', six were patients who developed cerebral vasospasm. This was due to the initial disease, rather than a complication of the procedure itself.

Postmortem examinations

Key Point

- *Two out of seven postmortem examinations did not confirm the clinical team's impression; it is for this reason that more postmortem examinations are recommended.*

Twenty-eight of the 36 deaths were reported to the coroner and of these three had a coroner's postmortem performed. Of the remaining 33 cases, only six patients had a hospital postmortem. Of the nine postmortems performed, a radiologist attended in seven cases. The team received a copy of the postmortem report in six of the nine cases.

Question 2.2: Did the pathological information confirm the team's clinical impression?

Yes	5
No	2
Not answered	2
Total	9

Table 2.9: Specialty of the pathologist who performed the postmortem examination	
Specialty	**Number**
General histopathologist	4
Neuropathologist	3
Home Office histopathologist	1
Not answered	1
Total	**9**

The postmortem rate was low, though slightly higher than for surgical specialties previously cited by NCEPOD[18]. The attendance of radiologists was commendable. It is interesting that in two out of seven cases the postmortem did not confirm the team's clinical impression:

CASE 4 • *A 36-year-old patient had a GDC to a large berry aneurysm of the internal carotid artery. She developed a cerebral thrombosis from which she died. The neuroradiologist thought the coil had impinged on the lumen of the internal carotid artery, but the postmortem showed it was in perfect position.*

CASE 5 • *A 57-year-old patient had an uncomplicated embolisation of an anterior communicating aneurysm which had bled. He was allowed home a week later but was readmitted after two days with confusion and agitation. It was thought that the coil had prolapsed back into the parent vessel although a CT scan showed no focal ischaemia. He deteriorated and died and postmortem showed death was caused by acute pulmonary oedema due to coronary artery disease.*

These cases illustrate the reason why postmortems are recommended.

Specialist neuropathologists are few in number and it is not surprising that they only performed a third of the postmortems; ideally they should be doing the majority.

AUDIT AND QUALITY

Audit

In 22/36 (61%) cases the death was discussed at an audit meeting; it was felt that all should be considered, highlighting those to be discussed in detail.

Quality of questionnaires

A case summary was written in 34/36 (94%) questionnaires returned. In 33 the general standard of filling in the forms was good; a further two were felt to be fair and one mediocre. None were considered to be really poor.

Standard of care

In 34/36 (94%) cases the standard of care was felt to be adequate and appropriate. In two cases there was cause for concern. One was a patient who had endovascular coiling for a subarachnoid haemorrhage, developed postprocedure vasospasm and whose general condition was deteriorating; there was no ICU or HDU bed and this lack was felt to contribute to the death of the patient.

The other was an overweight patient having embolisation of an aneurysm who developed a serious groin haematoma. There was a delay in recognising this and during the subsequent surgical repair of the femoral artery the patient suffered hypovolaemia which caused an exaggeration of the cerebral state. The use of newer arterial closure devices to secure haemostasis after femoral puncture should be considered in patients at a high risk of serious groin haematoma[19]. It is obviously important that the staff caring for these patients are aware of the risk of groin haematoma and should be observing carefully for it so that appropriate timely treatment can be given.

REFERENCES

1. *Report of the working party on guidelines for sedation by non-anaesthetists.* Royal College of Surgeons of England. London, 1993.

2. Berridge DC, Niakin GS, Hopkinson BR. *Local low-dose intra-arterial thrombolytic therapy, the risks of major stroke and haemorrhage.* Br J Surg, 1989; **76**:1230-1232.

3. Dawson K, Armon M, Braithwaite B, Galland R, Kendrick R, Downes M, Earnshaw JJ, Hamilton G. *Stroke during intra-arterial thrombolysis: a survey of experience in the UK.* Br J Surg, 1996; **83**:568.

4. Braithwaite BD, Davies B, Birch PA, Heather BP, Earnshaw JJ. *Management of acute leg ischaemia in the elderly.* Br J Surg, 1998; **85**: 217-220.

5. Working Party on Thrombolysis in the Management of Limb Ischaemia. *Thrombolysis in the Management of Lower Limb Peripheral Arterial Occlusion - A consensus document.* Am J Cardiol, 1998; **81**: 207-218.

6. Allermand H, Westergaard-Nielsen J, Neilsen OS. *Lower limb embolectomy in old age.* J Cardiovasc Surg, 1986; **27**: 440-2.

7. Valji K, Bookstein JJ, Roberts AC, Sanchez RB. *Occluded peripheral arteries and bypass grafts: stagnation as an end point for pulse-spray pharmacomechanical thrombolysis.* Radiology, 1993; **188**: 389-394.

8. Allison D, Wallace S. In: *Diagnostic Radiology: a Textbook of Medical Imaging.* Eds. Grainger and Allison. Churchill Livingstone, 1997; 3rd edition. **3**: 2525-2550.

9. Nicholson AA, Ettles DF, Arnold A, Greenstone M, Dyet JF. *Treatment of Malignant Superior Vena Caval Obstruction: Metal Stents or Radiation Therapy?* JVIR, 1997; **8**: 781-785.

10. Dick R, Patch D, Clarke D. *Who's for Tips?* Clinical Radiology, 1995; **50**: 590-592.

11. Tibballs JM, Patch D, Watkinson AF, Dick R. *Transjugular Intrahepatic Portosystemic Shunt: Indications, Techniques, Complications and Outcomes.* Interventional Radiology Monitor, 1997; **1**: 47-54.

12. Thromboembolic risk factors (THRIFT) consensus group. *Risk of, and prophylaxis for, venous thromboembolism in hospital patients.* BMJ, 1992; **305**: 567-574.

13. Guglielmi G, Vinuela F, Duckwiler G, et al. *Endovascular treatment of posterior circulation aneurysms by electrothrombosis using electrically detachable coils.* J Neursurg, 1992; **77**: 515-524.

14. Guglielmi G. *Embolization of Intracranial Aneurysms with Detachable Coils and Electrothrombosis.* In: *Interventional Neuroradiology.* Eds. Vinuela F, Halbach V, Dion J. Raven Press, 1992; 63-75.

15. Kassell NF, Torner JC, Hale EC et al. *The international cooperative study on the timing of aneurysm surgery. Part 1: Overall management results.* Journal of Neurosurgery, 1990; **73**: 18-36.

16. Gallimore SC, Hoile RW, Ingram GS, Sherry KM. *The Report of the National Confidential Enquiry into Perioperative Deaths 1994/95.* London, 1997.

17. Alvord EC, Loeser JD, Bailey W, Copass MK. *Subarachnoid haemorrhage due to ruptured aneurysm. A simple method of estimating prognosis.* Archives of Neurology, 1972; **27**: 273-284.

18. Gray AJG, Hoile RW, Ingram GS, Sherry KM. *The Report of the National Confidential Enquiry into Perioperative Deaths 1996/97.* London, 1998.

19. Beyer-Enke SA, Soldner J, Zeitler E. *Immediate sealing of arterial puncture site following femoropopliteal angioplasty: a prospective randomised trial.* Cardiovasc. Interven. Radiol, 1996; **19**: 406-410.

References

APPENDIX A - ABBREVIATIONS

A&E .... Accident & Emergency

ACT .... Activated clotting time

ASA .... American Society of Anesthesiologists

AV .... Arteriovenous

AVM .... Arteriovenous malformation

CC .... Caroticocavernous

CCST .... Certificate of Completion
of Specialist Training

CNS .... Central nervous system

CT .... Computerised tomography

DVT .... Deep vein thrombosis

ECG .... Electrocardiogram

GCS .... Glasgow coma scale

GDC .... Guglielmi detachable coil

HDU .... High dependency unit

ICU .... Intensive care unit

IVC .... Inferior vena cava

SAH .... Subarachnoid haemorrhage

SHO .... Senior house officer

SpR .... Specialist registrar

SVC .... Superior vena cava

THRIFT .... Thromboembolic risk factors

TIPS .... Transjugular intrahepatic portosystemic
shunt

WFNS .... World Federation of Neurological
Surgeons

Appendices

APPENDIX B - NCEPOD
CORPORATE STRUCTURE

The National Confidential Enquiry into Perioperative Deaths (NCEPOD) is an independent body to which a corporate commitment has been made by the Associations, Colleges and Faculties related to its areas of activity. Each of these bodies nominates members of the Steering Group.

Steering Group

(as at 1 October 2000)

Chairman
Mr John Ll Williams

Members
Mrs M Beck   *(Royal College of Ophthalmologists)*

Dr J F Dyet   *(Royal College of Radiologists)*

Dr H H Gray   *(Royal College of Physicians of London)*

Dr P Kishore   *(Faculty of Public Health Medicine)*

Mr G T Layer   *(Association of Surgeons of Great Britain and Ireland)*

Professor V J Lund   *(Royal College of Surgeons of England)*

Dr J M Millar   *(Royal College of Anaesthetists)*

Dr A J Mortimer   *(Royal College of Anaesthetists)*

Professor J H Shepherd *(Royal College of Obstetricians and Gynaecologists)*

Dr P J Simpson   *(Royal College of Anaesthetists)*

Mr M F Sullivan   *(Royal College of Surgeons of England)*

Professor P G Toner   *(Royal College of Pathologists)*

Professor T Treasure   *(Royal College of Surgeons of England)*

Dr D J Wilkinson   *(Association of Anaesthetists of Great Britain and Ireland)*

Mr J Ll Williams   *(Faculty of Dental Surgery, Royal College of Surgeons of England)*

Observers
Mr P Milligan   *(Institute of Health Services Management)*

Dr P A Knapman   *(Coroners' Society of England and Wales)*

NCEPOD is a company limited by guarantee, and a registered charity, managed by Trustees.

Trustees

Chairman	Mr J Ll Williams
Treasurer	Dr J N Lunn
	Dr J Lumley
	Dr P J Simpson
	Mr M F Sullivan

Clinical Coordinators

The Steering Group appoint the Principal Clinical Coordinators for a defined tenure. The Principal Clinical Coordinators lead the review of the data relating to the annual sample, advise the Steering Group and write the reports. They may also from time to time appoint Clinical Coordinators, who must be engaged in active academic/clinical practice (in the NHS) during the full term of office.

Principal Clinical Coordinators

Anaesthesia	Dr G S Ingram
Surgery	Mr R W Hoile

Clinical Coordinators

Anaesthesia	Dr A J G Gray
	Dr K M Sherry
Surgery	Mr K G Callum
	Mr I C Martin

Appendices

Funding

The total annual cost of NCEPOD is approximately £500,000 (1999/2000). We are pleased to acknowledge the support of the following, who contributed to funding the Enquiry in 1999/2000.

National Institute for Clinical Excellence
Welsh Office
Health and Social Services Executive (Northern Ireland)
States of Guernsey Board of Health
States of Jersey
Department of Health and Social Security, Isle of Man Government
Aspen Healthcare
BMI Healthcare
BUPA
Community Hospitals Group
Nuffield Hospitals
PPP/Columbia Healthcare
Benenden Hospital
King Edward VII Hospital, Midhurst
King Edward VII's Hospital for Officers, London
St Martin's Hospitals
The Heart Hospital
The London Clinic

This funding covers the total cost of the Enquiry, including administrative salaries and reimbursements for Clinical Coordinators, office accommodation charges, computer and other equipment as well as travelling and other expenses for the Coordinators, Steering Group and advisory groups.

Appendices

Appendix C - Data Collection and Review Methods

The National Confidential Enquiry into Perioperative Deaths (NCEPOD) reviews clinical practice and aims to identify remediable factors in the practice of anaesthesia, all types of surgery and other invasive procedures. The Enquiry considers the quality of the delivery of care and not specifically causation of death. The commentary in the reports is based on peer review of the data, questionnaires and notes submitted; it is not a research study based on differences against a control population, and does not attempt to produce any kind of comparison between clinicians or hospitals.

The concept of one-year studies reviewing interventional vascular and neurovascular radiological procedures represented a unique opportunity for collaboration between NCEPOD and the Royal College of Radiologists. The studies were also the first by NCEPOD to specifically collect denominator data on the total number of procedures performed.

The data collection and review methods common to the two studies are described below.

Scope

All National Health Service hospitals carrying out interventional radiology procedures in England, Scotland, Wales and Northern Ireland, and public hospitals in Guernsey and Jersey were invited to participate in the studies.

The period for which data was collected ran from 1 April 1998 to 31 March 1999 and participation was voluntary, being before the introduction of clinical governance and any requirement to take part in this type of Enquiry.

Data collection and review

Hospitals were invited, via the Director of Radiology, to participate in the study and to nominate a suitable person to take responsibility for submission of the necessary data. The names of those who agreed to undertake this task are shown in Appendices D and E, and were predominantly consultant radiologists.

Participating hospitals were asked to submit aggregated data on the total number of patients undergoing radiological procedures on a monthly basis. In addition, information was requested on any patient who died in hospital within 30 days of the procedure. If hospitals were aware of deaths occurring at home, they were invited to report these as well.

Review of deaths

For every case where NCEPOD was informed of a death within 30 days of the procedure, a questionnaire was sent to the relevant consultant radiologist. A copy of the full questionnaire is available from NCEPOD on request. The questionnaires were identified only by a number, allocated in the NCEPOD office. Copies of procedure notes, X-ray reports, postmortem notes and histology reports were also requested.

Data analysis

The NCEPOD administrative staff managed the collection, recording and analysis of data. The data were aggregated to produce the tables and information in the report.

Advisory groups

The designated NCEPOD Clinical Coordinator (K Callum), together with the advisory group members whose names are shown at the front of this report, reviewed the completed questionnaires and the aggregated data.

Confidentiality

NCEPOD is registered with the Data Protection Registrar and abides by the Data Protection Principles. All reporting forms, questionnaires and other paper records are shredded once an individual report is ready for publication. Similarly, all identifiable data are removed from the computer database.

Before review of questionnaires by the Clinical Coordinators or any of the advisors, all identification is removed from the questionnaires and accompanying papers. The source of the information is not revealed to any of the Coordinators or advisors.

NATIONAL CEPOD

Appendices

APPENDIX D - LOCAL REPORTERS

Interventional vascular radiology

Hospitals are listed according to regional divisions in place at the publication date. It should be noted that regional boundaries have changed since the 1998/99 data collection period described in this report.

Eastern

Bedford Hospital .... Dr R A Moxon

Norfolk & Norwich Hospital .... Ms M Gracie

Peterborough District Hospital .... Dr R E Moshy

Queen Elizabeth Hospital .... Dr M Sparks

Watford General Hospital .... Dr N Damani

West Suffolk Hospital .... Dr R J Godwin

London

Chelsea & Westminster Hospital .... Dr J McCall

Edgware General Hospital .... Dr K Lotzof

Epsom General Hospital .... Dr C D George

Farnborough Hospital .... Dr R Carver

Greenwich District Hospital .... Dr R Nagendran

Hammersmith Hospital ...... Professor A Hemingway

Hillingdon Hospital .... Dr N Chetty

Kingston Hospital .... Dr G Picken

Northwick Park Hospital .... Dr R Wilkins

Oldchurch Hospital .... Mrs A Deterville

St Bartholomew's Hospital .... Dr C Blakeney

St Helier Hospital.......................... Dr E A North

St Mary's Hospital.......................... Dr R Morgan

St Thomas' Hospital .... Dr A Irvine

The Middlesex Hospital .... Dr M J Raphael

University Hospital Lewisham .... Dr C Kennedy

West Middlesex University
Hospital .... Ms L Armistead

Whipps Cross Hospital .... Dr N Reading

North West

Alder Hey Children's Hospital .... Dr L Abernethy

Arrowe Park Hospital .... Dr M Lipton

Blackburn Royal Infirmary .... Ms P A Fenton

Chorley & South Ribble District
General Hospital .... Dr R C Stockwell

Countess of Chester Hospital .... Dr G T Abbott

Furness General Hospital .... Dr P J S Crawshaw

Halton General Hospital .... Dr G J Murphy

Leighton Hospital.......................... Dr S Zaman

Macclesfield District General
Hospital.............................. Dr C F Loughran

Manchester Royal Infirmary .... Dr N Chalmers

North Manchester General Hospital ...... Dr A N Khan

Royal Albert Edward Infirmary.......... Dr C L Poon

Royal Bolton Hospital.................... Dr J S Tuck

Royal Lancaster Infirmary .... Dr J M Lavelle

Royal Liverpool University Hospital ..... Dr D Gould

Royal Preston Hospital.................... Ms R Fowles

The Royal Oldham
Hospital.......................... Dr L L K Lee Cheong

The Victoria Hospital .... Dr R W Bury

University Hospital, Aintree .... Dr E A O'Grady

Warrington Hospital .... Dr J McCaig

Withington Hospital .... Dr R Ashleigh

Northern & Yorkshire

Bradford Royal Infirmary .... Dr S Chakraverty

Cumberland Infirmary .... Dr G Athey

Darlington Memorial Hospital ..... Dr R G Henderson

Freeman Hospital .... Dr R J T Owen

Friarage Hospital .... Dr J M Randall

Harrogate District Hospital .... Dr J Rose

Hartlepool General Hospital .... Dr G J Doyle

Huddersfield Royal Infirmary .... Dr R A Paes

Hull Royal Infirmary .... Dr J Dyet

Leeds General Infirmary .... Ms D Marriott

North Tees General Hospital .... Dr N P Tait

North Tyneside General
Hospital .... Dr A W Edirisooriya

Pinderfields General Hospital .... Mr G Holdsworth

Scarborough Hospital .... Dr I G H Renwick

South Cleveland Hospital .... Dr G Leen

South Tyneside District Hospital .... Dr L Cope

St James's University Hospital ...... Dr I Robertson

Sunderland Royal Hospital .... Dr S England

York District Hospital .... Mr A Magson

South East

Ashford Hospital .... Dr R Davies

Conquest Hospital .... Mrs K How

Eastbourne District General
Hospital .... Dr H Anderson

Frimley Park Hospital .... Ms S Connor

Kent & Canterbury Hospital .... Dr I D Morrison

Kettering General Hospital .... Dr S Peterson

Medway Maritime Hospital .... Dr K Reddy

Milton Keynes General Hospital ...... Dr A Ul-Haq

Northampton General Hospital ...... Dr R Kendrick

Princess Royal Hospital .... Dr I J Runcie

Queen Elizabeth the
Queen Mother Hospital .... Dr G Giancola

Royal Berkshire Hospital .... Dr E P H Torrie

Royal Hampshire County Hospital ..... Dr A C Page

Royal Sussex County Hospital .... Dr T N Doyle

Southampton General Hospital .... Dr A Odurny

St Peter's Hospital .... Dr M F Creagh

St Richard's Hospital .... Dr N S Ashford

Stoke Mandeville Hospital .... Dr R Bodley

The John Radcliffe Hospital .... Dr P Bordman

The North Hampshire Hospital .... Dr G Plant

Wexham Park Hospital .... Dr M Charig

William Harvey Hospital .... Mr P French

South West

Bristol Royal Infirmary .... Professor M R Rees

Cheltenham General Hospital .... Dr M Gibson

Derriford Hospital .... Dr C A Roobottom

Frenchay Hospital .... Dr M H Morse

Gloucestershire Royal Hospital .... Dr P A Birch

Princess Margaret Hospital .... Dr L K Jackson

Royal Bournemouth Hospital .... Dr Shepherd

Royal Cornwall Hospital .... Dr K S Blanshard

Royal Devon and Exeter Hospital ..... Dr C R Bayliss

Royal United Hospital .... Dr A Chalmers

Salisbury District Hospital .... Dr R A Frost

Taunton & Somerset Hospital .... Dr J Bell

Torbay District General Hospital .... Dr R H Fox

Yeovil District Hospital .... Dr N C G Bathurst

Trent

Barnsley District General Hospital .... Dr D Nag

Chesterfield & North Derbyshire
Royal Hospital .... Dr A Cohen

Derbyshire Royal Infirmary .... Dr D Hinwood

Diana Princess of Wales Hospital .... Dr R W J Harries

Doncaster Royal Infirmary .... Dr J Y Mackinlay

Glenfield Hospital .... Dr R Keal

King's Mill Hospital .... Dr P N Panto

Leicester General Hospital .... Ms M Turner

Leicester Royal Infirmary .... Dr G Fishwick

Lincoln County Hospital .... Dr C I Rothwell

Northern General Hospital .... Dr P A Gaines

Nottingham City Hospital .... Dr A R Manhire

Pilgrim Hospital .... Dr G M McGann

Rotherham District General
Hospital .... Dr P A Spencer

University Hospital, Nottingham ...... Dr R Gregson

West Midlands

Alexandra Hospital .... Dr C Phillips

Birmingham Children's Hospital .... Dr P John

Birmingham Heartlands Hospital ...... Dr P Crowe

Dudley Road Hospital .... Dr M S Moss

George Eliot Hospital .... Dr K A Vallance

Kidderminster General Hospital ...... Dr U L Udeshi

New Cross Hospital .... Dr M Collins

Princess Royal Hospital .... Dr R A Manns

Queen Elizabeth Hospital .... Dr S P Olliff

Queen's Hospital .... Dr K Nanda

Royal Shrewsbury Hospital .... Dr M R E Dean

Russells Hall Hospital .... Dr A P Wolinski

Sandwell General Hospital .... Dr J Leahy

Walsgrave Hospital .... Dr A Vohrah

Warwick Hospital .... Dr F Millard

Worcester Royal Infirmary .... Dr P L Slaney

Northern Ireland

Belfast City Hospital .... Dr L Johnston

Royal Victoria Hospital .... Dr P K Ellis

Scotland

Falkirk & District Royal Infirmary ...... Dr J E Barry

Gartnavel General Hospital .... Dr R D Edwards

Glasgow Royal Infirmary .... Dr A W Reid

Ninewells Hospital .... Dr J W Shaw

Queen Margaret Hospital .... Dr H Ireland

Raigmore Hospital .... Dr D M Nichols

Royal Hospital for Sick Children .... Dr A Maclennan

Royal Infirmary of Edinburgh ...... Dr G C McInnes

Victoria Infirmary .... Dr A C Downie

Wales

Morriston Hospital .... Dr D E Roberts

Neath General Hospital .... Dr D E Roberts

Nevill Hall Hospital .... Dr H Reed

Prince Philip Hospital .... Dr T N W Evans

Princess of Wales Hospital .... Dr W Tudor Young

Royal Glamorgan Hospital .... Dr E Hicks

Royal Gwent Hospital .... Dr B A Sullivan

University Hospital of Wales .... Dr A M Wood

Ysbyty Glan Clwyd .... Dr E H Moss

Ysbyty Gwynedd .... Dr P D Birch

Channel Islands

Princess Elizabeth Hospital,
Guernsey .... Dr J Hanaghan

Jersey General Hospital .... Dr A P Nisbet

APPENDIX E - LOCAL REPORTERS

Interventional neurovascular radiology

Hospitals are listed according to regional divisions in place at the publication date. It should be noted that regional boundaries have changed since the 1998/99 data collection period described in this report.

Eastern

Addenbrooke's Hospital .... Dr J N P Higgins

London

Atkinson Morley's Hospital .... Dr A Clifton

Charing Cross Hospital .... Dr I R Colquhoun

Great Ormond Street Hospital for Sick Children .... Dr W Taylor

King's College Hospital .... Dr M A Jeffree

Oldchurch Hospital .... Mrs A Deterville

The National Hospital for Neurology & Neurosurgery .... Dr W Taylor

The Royal Free Hospital .... Dr A R Valentine

The Royal London Hospital .... Dr P Butler

North West

Hope Hospital .... Dr D G Hughes

Manchester Royal Infirmary .... Dr R D Laitt

Walton Centre for Neurology & Neurosurgery .... Dr T Nixon

Northern & Yorkshire

Hull Royal Infirmary .... Dr C Rowland Hill

Leeds General Infirmary .... Dr M Nelson

Middlesbrough General Hospital .... Dr J Dervin

Newcastle General Hospital .... Dr A Gholkar

South East

Hurstwood Park Neurological Centre .... Dr J Olney

Radcliffe Infirmary .... Dr A J Molyneux

Southampton General Hospital .... Dr J Millar

South West

Frenchay Hospital .... Dr S A Renowden

Trent

Royal Hallamshire Hospital .... Dr T J Hodgson

University Hospital, Nottingham .... Dr T Jaspan

West Midlands

Queen Elizabeth Hospital .... Dr R West

Northern Ireland

Royal Victoria Hospital .... Dr H Kamel

Scotland

Southern General Hospital .... Dr J Bhattacharya

Western General Hospital .... Dr R Sellar

Wales

University Hospital of Wales .... Dr S Halpin

NATIONAL CEPOD 53

Appendices

APPENDIX F - PARTICIPANTS

Consultant vascular radiologists

The following consultant vascular radiologists returned at least one questionnaire relating to the period 1 April 1998 to 31 March 1999.

Abbott G.
Alcorn D.
Alner M.R.
Aref F.
Ashleigh R.A.
Banerjee A.
Birch P.A.
Birch P.D.
Blanshard K.S.
Bowker A.M.B.
Bruce D.
Cavanagh P.M.
Chakraverty S.
Chalmers A.H.
Chalmers N.
Charig M.
Cleveland T.
Cockburn J.F.
Cope L.H.
Corrigan N.
Crowe P.
D'Souza S.P.D.
Dacie J.E.
Denunzio M.C.
Downie A.C.
Doyle G.J.D.
Doyle T.N.
Dux A.E.W.
Dyet J.F.
Edwards R.
England S.J.P.
Ettles D.F.
Fairlie N.
Fawcitt R.A.
Ferrando J.R.
Fowler R.F.
Frost R.A.
Gaines P.A.
George C.D.
Giancola G.
Gibson J.M.
Girling S.D.
Godwin R.J.
Gould D.
Hacking N.
Hardman J.
Hartley R.
Hayward S.
Hinwood D.C.
Ignotus P.
Isaacs J.L.
Jackson L.K.

Jewell F.
Jeyagopal N.S.
Johnson K.J.
Keane A.
Kelly I.M.G.
Kendrick R.
Kennedy C.
Kinsella D.C.
Lakin K.L.H.
Lamb G.H.
Leahy J.F.
Lee Cheong L.
Leen G.
Loose H.W.C.
Lowe R.A.
Mackie G.
Malthouse S.
Marsh R.L.
McCall J.M.
McConnell C.A.
McGann G.
McInnes G.C.
McPherson S.J.
McWilliams R.G.
Mitchell A.
Morgan R.A.
Morrison I.D.
Moss J.
Moss M.S.
Murphy G.J.
Nagendran R.
Newland C.N.
Nicholson A.A.
Odurny A.
Olliff S.P.
Owen M.
Owen R.O.
Page A.C.
Panto P.N.
Pelling M.
Peterson S.
Phillips-Hughes J.P.H.
Plant G.
Procter A.E.
Raphael M.J.
Redhead D.
Reed D.H.
Renny F.H.B.
Roberts D.
Roobottom C.A.R.
Rose J.D.G.
Runcie I.

Sampson C.
Scally J.
Scott-Barrett S.
Seymour R.
Shepherd D.F.C.
Singanayagam J.K.
Sissons G.
Smith W.H.
Sparks M.J.
Spencer P.A.
Stockwell R.C.
Sullivan B.A.
Tawn J.
Thavia V.R.
Thomas H.G.T.
Tottle A.J.
Toye R.
Tuck J.S.
Turner P.J.
Tuson J.
Vohrah A.R.
Walter D.F.
Watkin E.M.
Wells I.P.
West R.J.
Williams J.G.
Wood A.M.
Young W.T

NATIONAL CEPOD

APPENDIX G - PARTICIPANTS

Consultant neurovascular radiologists

The following consultant neurovascular radiologists returned at least one questionnaire relating to the period 1 April 1998 to 31 March 1999.

Bartlett R.J.V.
Bhattacharya J.J.
Buckenham T.
Byrne J.V.
Clifton A.G.
Dervin J.E.
Gholkar A.
Halpin S.F.S.
Higgins J.N.P.
Hodgson T.J.
Hughes D.
Jaspan T.
McConachie N.S.
McKinstry S.
Molyneux A.J.
O'Sullivan M.
Rowland Hill C.A.
Sellar R.
Teasdale E.